BREAK
THE CODE
OF YOUR
ILLNESS

BREAK
THE CODE
OF YOUR
ILLNESS

The Link Between Emotional Distress and Health Disorders

ISABELLE BENAROUS

Bioreprogramming® Press

LOS ANGELES, CALIFORNIA

1st printing August 2010 • 2nd printing 2011 • 3rd printing 2012

ISBN: 978-0-9829157-0-7
LCCN: 2010911723

ATTENTION CORPORATIONS, UNIVERSITIES, COLLEGES, AND PRO-FESSIONAL ORGANIZATIONS: Quantity discounts are available on bulk purchases of this book for educational, gift purposes, or as premiums for increasing magazine subscriptions or renewals. Special books or book excerpts can also be created to fit specific needs. For information, please contact Bioreprogramming® Press; email: info@bioreprogramming.net; phone: 323-717-6107.

www.bioreprogramming.net

To Tony

CONTENTS

INTRODUCTION

My name is Isabelle Benarous. I am an NLP (Neuro Linguistic Programming) trainer, specializing in the resolution of emotional conflicts related to disease. I created this book to share with you important knowledge about the origin of illness, particularly cancer.

Individuals who healed from cancer are all around us, and we know they are the exceptions that challenge traditional medical theories and statistics. If there is an exception to a theory, it means the theory is not fully correct. This observation is what motivated my quest for answers, when a loved one was unexpectedly diagnosed with stage-four lung cancer in 2000. What were those exceptions about? What did it take to become an exception and how could anyone in the medical field deny this possibility? That was what I needed to know and that's how my journey began, through intensive study of German New Medicine® and Total Biology®, which I believe have collectively uncovered the origin of illness.

After the loved one became "an exception" I was determined to dedicate myself to this type of approach and subsequently specialized in the resolution of emotional distress. The origin of cancer as well as other illnesses has been exposed and these findings need to be known and accessible to the public. Over the past ten years, I successfully helped numerous individuals resolve their emotional conflicts, and in the process I developed the Bioreprogramming® method. This method focuses on decoding the origin of conflicts related to illness and offers powerful techniques for solving emotional distress.

The purpose of this book is to give you the opportunity to look at disease with a new awareness. It will also provide health practitioners and students of the Bioreprogramming® method with a summary describing the findings of Dr. Hamer, called German New Medicine®, as well as the concept of Total Biology® developed by Dr. Claude Sabbah. The following writings represent an introduction to a new approach that will in the years to come revolutionize the world's vision about the origin of disease. The reader needs to be aware that the information described within this document is very condensed. This approach, which is in constant evolution, contains complex biological ramifications, and the premises offered in this book should be integrated with open-mindedness.

While you are reading this document you might oscillate between old and new belief systems regarding health, life, and evolution. You may consider giving yourself time to evaluate these new findings, observe your life through a new lens, and explore new possibilities.

This knowledge has changed my life and the lives of many others, and it can also change yours as you realize you have the power and ability to create your own healing. I am blessed to be able to share this life changing information with you.

Disclaimer

The information presented in this document should only be used as a guide for educational purposes regarding the origin of disease. It is not intended to replace the recommendations of a licensed health practitioner or any medical intervention.

THE STORY OF JULIA

On a bright sundrenched morning, Julia was in her kitchen preparing breakfast for herself and her husband Richard. She was in a particularly cheerful mood because her best friend of twenty-five years was getting married for the first time later that day at the age of forty-one.

When Richard came in the kitchen and sat at the table, Julia noticed that he was on edge and somewhat disconnected, eating his meal without uttering a word. When she asked if he had slept well, he shook his head "no." Julia did not say anything. She would not allow Richard's bad mood to spoil her day.

After breakfast, Richard went back into the bedroom. Julia thought he went back to bed. However, an hour later he appeared carrying a small suitcase and his coat and simply said, *"Julia, I am leaving you. I will never come back. Please don't ask me why. I am leaving now."*

As he headed out the door, Julia ran after him screaming his name, but he would not stop. He did not even acknowledge her. Julia was stunned, speechless, caught off guard, and felt as if the ground had been ripped away from beneath her feet. Her husband was leaving her. This whole incident made no sense to Julia. She thought they were a fine couple; they seemed happy and she was not aware of any specific problems. During her five-year marriage to Richard, she had been very loving, selflessly caring, and nurturing toward him.

As she sat in the open doorway watching Richard drive away, she was trembling uncontrollably, her heart was pounding so hard it felt it would explode out of her chest; she could not catch her breath; she could not even cry; she felt nauseated. For Julia, time had stopped. After twenty minutes of feeling stunned, cold, and unable to move, she gathered all her strength to get up, slowly walk back inside the house, and collapse on the bed.

She did not go to her friend's wedding that afternoon. Instead she spent the time repeatedly calling Richard's cell phone, with no response. As days went by, all efforts to reach him were in vain. Richard had quit his job and disappeared. His family and friends told Julia that they did not know where he was. She was very confused and also worried for Richard's well-being.

Six months later, she had signed the divorce papers Richard's lawyer had sent her and wanted to put this experience behind her. She now had something more important to take care of: her health. During a routine exam, Julia found out she had a malignant tumor in her right breast. It was the first time anyone had been diagnosed with breast cancer in her family. She was only forty-two years old, did not smoke or drink, did not live a sedentary life, was not overweight, and had never used birth control pills. On the contrary, Julia ate healthy organic food, exercised regularly, drank plenty of water, and every day breathed fresh country air during her morning jogs in the Vincennes woods just outside of Paris.

What had happened to Julia? Bad luck? How is it possible that suddenly, at age forty-two, cells in Julia's breast mutated and formed a tumor? Why now and not a year before or two years before that or even a year or two later? What an awful year it had been for Julia! Everything seemed to happen at the same time. She felt her life was falling apart and it made no sense to her. Or maybe it did make sense. Could Julia's disease be related to the only element that was out of the ordinary that year? Her husband had left one morning without an explanation and never came back. This was an enormous event and a major shock for Julia. Her emotional distress felt similar to the one she had experienced thirty-six years ago, at the age of six years old, when her father left the house after a fight with Julia's mother on their wedding anniversary. He stormed out of the house and said he was never coming back. Julia loved and cared about her dad very much. Julia ran after him, screaming for him not to go. He came back three days later, with a hangover, and stayed with Julia's mom for another fifteen years before he died.

The incident with her father represented a traumatic event for Julia, and although buried in her past, it was still part of her history. Julia's story illustrates how our subconscious mind can store away our memories and how nothing is ever emotionally forgotten. Each experience has a specific feeling attached to it, which is called the "felt experience." As we go through life, we subconsciously link together emotional states of the same type. Our brain recalls experiences from our past that resurface in our present each time we go through emotions of the same nature.

For instance, when Julia's husband left her unexpectedly, it triggered an unconscious association in her mind of when her father suddenly left her family. The emotion she felt at six years old was an unconscious stress that resurfaced with the sudden departure of her husband Richard. As observed by Carl Gustav Jung, "Everything that does not rise into consciousness comes back as destiny."

The way Julia worried about her father for three painful days when she was six was the same way she now worried about Richard. Only this time her concern continued for weeks. How long was Richard going to stay away? Where was he going to sleep? How could she know if he was going to be safe? Did he leave her for another woman? Maybe Richard was endangered by a mental illness or perhaps he was having an identity crisis. She wanted to be there for him, help him, comfort him. For several days, Julia could not eat or sleep normally. Her imagination was constantly at work and her mind on high alert as she looked for answers to alleviate her stress. No matter what the reasons were that prompted Richard to leave, she wanted him to come back so that she could take care of him and make everything better. More than anything, Julia was consumed by her maternal instinct.

Symbolically, the specific organ an individual associates with nurturing is the breast, whose role is to produce milk. In a broad sense, a concern related to anyone or anything a woman wants to mother and protect, is called a "nest-worry conflict." Julia's extreme emotional distress about Richard leaving unexpectedly found its expression in her breast tissue. Subconsciously, Julia's brain triggered a manifestation in her body, soliciting precisely the organ corresponding to her "felt experience."

Six years later, Julia had overcome the illness and, although she had met another man, she had not remarried. She found out through an old friend that Richard was living in his hometown in northern France and he did not want to have any contact with her. This was fine with Julia. She was now living a peaceful life; she liked her job and was happy with her boyfriend. She had stopped thinking of Richard and felt free.

Some years later, she got invited to the wedding of the daughter of a long time friend. It was a big wedding with over a hundred guests. After the church ceremony, everyone gathered at a fancy restaurant for the reception. Julia sat at a table with her boyfriend and a couple of old friends. Suddenly, she noticed Richard in the crowd of guests. She stood up and started to walk towards him. The second Richard saw her, he turned away and left the room before she could reach him. Julia was speechless, caught off guard, and shocked. At that moment, the past experiences and their related emotional stresses resurfaced in Julia's mind.

Julia's emotional history was re-awakened when she saw Richard, and for an instant, she felt exactly the same way she did six years ago when he left. As a result, an immediate response to her emotional distress manifested. Her brain re-triggered the cellular memory related to nurturing, turning on the genes in her breast tissue responsible for the growth of a tumor. Five months after she saw Richard at the wedding, Julia's mammogram showed a "recurrence" of her cancer.

I met Julia in 2003. She wanted to learn more about the new approach regarding illness, which I will outline in this book. Julia was undergoing cancer treatment for the second time in her life. As she told me her story, we connected the two offsets of her illness with their emotional triggers. The revelation of the intimate link between her emotional life and her illness permitted Julia to recognize and unlock the subconscious stress directly related to the disease in her body. During that first meeting, tears of relief ran down her cheeks. For the first time since the beginning of her journey with cancer, everything made sense to Julia.

While Julia was continuing medical treatment, I saw her a few more times. She was able to achieve several personal breakthroughs as we worked on changing the limiting beliefs and perceptions rooted to her emotional distress. Although a bleak cancer prognosis had been given to her, the illness resolved, and she is cancer free to this day.

The Discovery

German New Medicine

A sudden, dramatic, personal tragedy led Dr. Ryke Geerd Hamer, formerly of the Universities of Munich and Tubingen in Germany, to a premise he called German New Medicine. This new approach resulted from a set of findings linking the nature of disease on universal biological principles and on the interaction between the three levels that make up the human organism: the psyche, the brain, and the organ. It culminated in Dr. Hamer's conviction that diseases have a biological meaning and are not mistakes of nature.

It was indeed a terrible mistake that caused the death of Dr. Hamer's 17-year-old son Dirk, who was accidentally shot while on a boat anchored off the Mediterranean island of Cavallo. It was August of 1978 when Vittorio Emanuele—the unofficial Prince of Naples and a somewhat controversial figure—was moored in his luxury yacht nearby and discharged his military rifle at someone who was attempting to steal a dinghy. He missed the thief and seriously injured Dirk Hamer, an innocent victim who never recovered from his injuries and died four months later.

Shortly after losing his son, Dr. Hamer was diagnosed with testicular cancer. Considering he had been healthy all his life, he suspected there might be a connection between the traumatic event of the death of his son and the onset of his illness. Later on, when he became head internist of an oncology clinic in Munich, Dr. Hamer decided to seek verification of his hypothesis by investigating traumas in the lives of his patients prior to a cancer diagnosis. Interestingly, he found that his cancer patients had experienced a deeply felt trauma a few months before the existence of their disease, and his observation is now supported by more than 40,000 cases. Dr. Hamer's findings have instigated a revolutionary approach to disease, especially regarding cancer, which was considered cellular anarchy up until his discovery enlightened our minds about the extraordinary meaning of illness.

Dirk Hamer Syndrome

After extensive research of thousands of patients, Dr. Hamer concluded that every cancer or cancer-like disease is the consequence of a sudden, dramatic, highly acute, isolating shock, which he called DHS (Dirk Hamer Syndrome), in honor of his son, whose death he believes led him to the discovery of the German New Medicine. This biological conflict-shock seems to cause the appearance of a focus of activity in the brain—called an "HH" (Hamerschenherd). This set of concentric rings (HH) is centered on a precise point of the brain and can be seen in a computerized tomography scan (CT).

In essence, each organ in the body has a function and is connected to a specific group of neurons in the brain that monitors the cells within that particular organ. Therefore, our brain controls the behavior of our cells. So when a human being is experiencing a state of intense stress, the brain has the capacity to prompt an adaptive response to alleviate it. Such response will generate a modification in the brain—an "HH"—and the organ controlled by that specific brain relay will then register a functional transformation, which directly corresponds to the way an experience is perceived and ultimately "felt" by an individual. This transformation in the body can manifest as a growth, as tissue loss, or as a loss of function.

It can be seen, then, that the experience of shock is simultaneous on three levels: the *psyche*, the *brain*, and the *organ*.

- The *psyche* expresses the meaning of the traumatic event—the so-called "conflict"—whether real, imaginary, symbolic, or virtual.
- The *brain* expresses the location of the disease (the "HH") where the isolation of a group of neurons and their alteration will take place, and communicates with the correlated organ, manufacturing a cellular change.
- The *organ* will express the biological meaning of the "conflict" according to the type of embryonic layer to which it is connected, and a change will manifest at a cellular level in the body.

Biological Response

Dr. Hamer advocates that illness is the direct result of a psychological conflict. Under this model, when a conflict generating extreme stress within an individual is not resolved, the brain will order a specific biological response in the body that will express the emotional struggle. Apparently the brain alleviates unmanageable stresses by expressing solutions to conflicts within our biology.

As human beings, we define our emotional struggles in a literal or figurative sense, subconsciously using primal language and animalistic sets of representations and emotions. Our perception of an experience will awaken our primary visceral maps, which connect our internal sensations with their corresponding organs. We might consider an experience to be "disgusting" (which corresponds to the colon), "suffocating" (lung), "staining" (skin dimension), "stinking" (sinuses), "indigestible" (stomach), and so on. An individual's verbal expression and description of an experience has a high significance. When individuals express their emotional stress, information can be gathered about the "felt sense" of their traumatic experience.

If we imagine four women going through the same sudden isolating traumatic shock, such as unexpected news that their child has a life-threatening illness, we may wonder why they do not all emotionally respond to the news in the same way or manifest the same disease. It is important, therefore, to understand the notion of "felt experience."

Each of us has a different way of giving meaning to our experiences, even though we all experience the world through the same five senses. What will determine our perception of the environment, and the resultant emotion towards a traumatic event, resides within the depth of our subconscious mind, which contains our life story, imprints and memories from the past, decisions made, values adopted, traditions, religions, upbringing, gestation programs, and ancestral mental maps.

We filter the environment in a way that permits us to succeed at waking up our latent conflicts, for which we have a subconscious affinity and a need to liberate. Our distortions about the environment are often proportional to the limitations experienced by the previous generations and by ourselves as we were growing up, lacking choices and resources that would permit us to see life differently. We are predisposed to our perceptions and illnesses through more ways than just the obvious ones.

In the example involving the four women, if the first woman perceives the situation about her child's health as a "nest-worry conflict," (which refers to a mother-child or a daughter-mother conflict), her emotional response might manifest a cell proliferation in her left or right mammary gland, due to the subconscious yearning to produce more milk to nurture her child. Whether she is innately right-handed or left-handed will determine which mammary gland will be affected.

Instinctively, a right-handed woman will hold her child in her left arm and feed the child with her left breast, thus permitting her right arm to be free, operational and able to deflect danger. In this case, a "nest-worry conflict" will affect the left breast. The right breast (for right-handed women) is linked to concerns regarding someone or something, which is mothered secondarily, such as a partner (*à la* Julia), family member, friend, pet, or object. This condition would be reversed and occur in the right breast for a left-handed woman.

The second woman may be a person with strong religious principles who has spent her life following the Bible and "making sacrifices" for God. In this particular case, the woman feels extremely angry with God after receiving the news that her child is sick and cannot "digest" the fact that He is making her child suffer. She feels betrayed, and her incapacity to process what she considers to be a "filthy morsel" (the injustice of God) might subsequently lead to a tumor in the colon. The tumor will function to produce more mucus to figuratively slide away the "morsel" towards the outside.

The third woman's perception may be an actual "death-fright" as she imagines that her child could stop breathing and die. Symbolically, she might want to take in more air for her child. Since staying alive is primarily linked to breathing and the lung's capacity to process oxygen, the alveoli of the lung would be the targeted organ in this case. A proliferation of cells in the alveoli allows for a greater oxygen exchange, thus resulting in lung cancer.

The fourth woman may have a strong belief system and inner resources permitting her to handle the situation with much less emotional stress than the three women mentioned above. For example, she might believe that her child is protected, no matter how bad the circumstances may seem. She may have an inherent, fervent, spiritual acceptance about life's challenges and their purpose—a perception that the presence of disease or even death is meant to engender spiritual growth. The example of the fourth woman shows how a difference in perception of a particular situation can prevent unmanageable stress. It is very possible that the fourth woman will remain free from any disease or symptoms related to her challenge.

Diseases are not triggered by circumstances but by ways of perception. Our thoughts, brain, and body do not operate independently. The synchronicity between the three is the key to understanding this new approach.

The Human Being

The Psyche

The human psyche (conscious mind) collects information from the outside world through the five senses (sight, sound, taste, smell, and touch). When an event occurs, individuals create a personalized evaluation in agreement with their values and belief system. Thereafter, their brain will adapt to the experience in accordance to their perception and emotional state. When individuals reason, they are under the illusion that they can make decisions and direct their life using their logic. In fact, we will see later on that the meanings given to our experiences and the decisions made are based on subconscious programs that influence the interpretations of the situations humans encounter in life.

The Brain

The brain is both a computer and a recorder, capable of processing about 20 million environmental stimuli per second. It permanently stays alert to our surroundings and filters the information we gather at conscious and subconscious levels. Subconsciously, we absorb without judgment the opinion that is formed and accepted by our conscious mind. Our brain has been molded by evolution to maintain the survival of the individual and the genetic progeny. It is simultaneously maintaining external and internal awareness, whether it is the blinking of an eye to avoid a projectile or the monitoring of our heart rate during exercise. Our brain will always operate in the present moment and control our behavioral and biological systems. It is autonomic, which means it configures and reconfigures itself in order to adapt to the environment, continually optimizing its abilities. The brain can be compared to a gigantic database of stored programs that contains our learned behaviors (walking, talking, writing, etc) as well as behaviors acquired since our birth from observing those around us (parents, peers, teachers, etc). It also contains built-in programs such as encoded memories we inherited from our ancestors and the programs we imprinted from our parents during gestation. Since we are not consciously aware of most of these programs, and therefore unable to modify them, our subconscious brain is running the show of our lives.

It is sometimes difficult to understand why our determination and focus are not sufficient enough to create the future we dream about. This is simply because our subconscious does not reason with the same type of logic as our conscious mind and it continues to follow its intrinsic imprints. It is quite similar to a machine that contains an immense load of pre-recorded tapes that are ready to play as soon as the appropriate environmental trigger presses the play button.

This process can be illustrated by certain animal experiments. For instance, as in humans, the presence of food activates the salivary glands in dogs. Pavlov conducted experimental work with laboratory dogs in which he rang a bell each time the dogs were fed. Over time, merely the sound of the bell without the presence of food elicited a salivary response in the dogs. An auditory trigger had conditioned the neurology of the dogs, and they were now programmed to elicit a biological reaction at the sound of a bell.

As human beings we have also undergone Pavlovian conditioning where our emotional states are accordingly induced by stimuli. What we see, hear, feel, smell, and taste are stored in our memory and become subconscious anchors as we experience life. We live in a world where millions of stimuli exist and can potentially trigger responses in our thinking, feeling, and reacting. Some of these triggers may affect us adversely.

For example, a man who has a severe allergic reaction every time he eats peanut butter may be triggering a childhood memory. At the age of five, he was eating a peanut butter sandwich when he experienced a trauma: After his mother hung up the phone in the kitchen, she told him that his beloved grandmother had just died of a heart attack. During the moment of such shock, the subconscious mind recorded at least one of the environmental components present at the time of the experience. In this case even a harmless substance such as peanut butter became associated with a shock. The subconscious mind programmed a strong allergic reaction to peanut butter, which is now associated with a conflict related to separation (loss of contact). Chronic allergies involve the epithelial tissues (primarily the skin). Any memory of a separation that has not been dealt with can be awakened by the stimulus of a component that is associated to the separation (in this case, the peanut butter). Our brain is capable of achieving very complex operations. However, it reacts to the environment in an almost simplistic fashion by creating survival metaphors such as food allergies. Our "felt experience" is guiding our brain to select the most appropriate response to protect us from stress.

Behavioral and biological responses are based on our reality (what is true to us) as well as our mental constructions (what we imagine). Our brain does not distinguish the difference between what we see externally and the images we create internally. It will react the same way to what is real, imaginary, virtual, or symbolic. Imagine a woman being awakened by an unusual noise in her house at four o'clock in the morning. She automatically thinks that burglars have broken into her home, and the images she manufactures in her mind will trigger a rush of adrenaline. As she goes down the stairs to investigate, she is anxious and afraid of what she might find, causing shortness of breath, a dry mouth, and trembling. Then she sees that the intruder is the neighbor's cat that has entered through an open window. The woman breathes a sigh of relief and immediately calms down. In this "fight or flight" situation, she has accepted both imaginary and real events as true and reacted accordingly on an emotional and biological level.

Two Sides of the Same Coin

Our conscious and subconscious minds rely upon each other in order to function. The conscious mind uses the resources of the subconscious, so that we don't have to relearn behaviors and can operate automatically. The autonomic brain gets information from the conscious mind and triggers responses to adapt to an ever-changing environment.

When we give meaning to our experiences as we process information from the outside world, we simultaneously engage in an emotional state. In order to be able to respond effectively to dangers in our environment, our brain will convert our gathered information into metaphors and symbols. This process permits our subconscious to immediately interpret the type of situation we are facing in order to activate the appropriate survival program.

A symbol or a metaphor can carry a maximum of information on a minimum of data. If I tell you that my friend Paul is like a "rock," you get an image of Paul without a detailed description. Because I used the word "rock" as a symbol, you might presuppose that Paul is a strong man, that he can withstand adversity, and that he is solid and reliable. Our subconscious brain is responsive to this form of communication because it saves time and energy, enabling a focus on biological monitoring and environmental dangers.

After gathering and analyzing the meaning of our thoughts, our brain acts independently from our consciousness, following its own trajectory in correlation with its blueprint. No matter how positive our conscious thoughts are, the power of our subconscious will prevail and override our conscious desires. For instance, a child who has been programmed to think he is worthless and does not deserve to be loved will carry a limiting imprint. Even though as an adult he realizes consciously his significance and repeats affirmations to convince himself otherwise, the fact remains that the deep imprint might persist, resulting in low self-esteem and eventually depression. Similarly, when an individual has a disease, positive affirmations often need to be supported by a subconscious de-programming of life-long accumulation of negative imprints and their related stresses.

The Body

The human body is made up of approximately a hundred trillion cells. Each cell works independently and for the entire body simultaneously, like an immense community. Every cell contributes to the survival of the entire organism by executing the programs transmitted by the brain. Internal receptors identify biological variations such as our heart rate, sugar levels, nutrient and hormonal levels and report them to the nervous system, which regulates metabolic function. External receptors are located almost everywhere throughout the body, reporting fluctuations in the environment, such as temperature, the humidity of the air, or the amount of light, so that the activity of our organs can be regulated accordingly.

Our nervous system maintains homeostasis, which is the balance of our body's basic functions. In case of a crisis in an organ, the brain will generate a solution in an attempt to re-establish proper functioning of the body. Observations of animals in their natural habitats may allow researchers to uncover the biological process behind the onset of certain so-called "diseases."

Biological Conflicts

The Story of a Fox

Animals can only experience conflicts, such as loss of offspring, fear of attack, or territorial threats, in real terms and not in imaginary, metaphorical, or virtual terms. For example a bird being kicked out of its nest by another bird represents a real territorial conflict as opposed to a human being who, when denied a favorite table at a restaurant, feels, symbolically, that their territory has been taken.

Accidents can happen in nature and animals often have the resources to overcome them. Dr. Hamer gives an example of a fox eating its prey rapidly (for example, a rabbit), for fear of it being stolen by other predators. If a big morsel composed of bone, nail, and fur travels down the digestive tract it may not be able to be broken down by regular digestion because of its size and composition. The morsel may therefore create a blockage in the stomach of the fox. Since there are no surgeons in nature, the fox would be able to survive for, at the most, three weeks. However, using its natural resources, the fox's body will create spasms and contractions in an attempt to regurgitate the morsel. If this process is not successful, the fox's brain will trigger another solution and launch a more suitable program to improve digestion and break down the morsel that is stuck. By programming a fast cell multiplication process, which creates a tumor in the mucosa of the stomach, a production of more digestive enzymes will take place, thus permitting an intense and rapid digestion. The brain provides the perfect solution to sustain life as long as possible in any given biological context. Once the morsel is

29

digested, the receptors in the stomach will inform the brain that the tumor is no longer necessary, thus resulting in its elimination. The above example seems to clearly suggest that cancer can be an intentional program of nature and in this case saved the life of the fox.

The Story of Frank

Frank is a small business owner, is married with two children, and owns a nice house in a good neighborhood. A couple of years ago, his best friend Rick went through a difficult divorce and lost everything, even his business. Because Rick was in such terrible financial shape, Frank hired him to work for his company. He also loaned him a substantial sum of money, which Rick used to rent an apartment and pay numerous debts he had accumulated during his divorce. The two men had been friends since childhood, and Frank felt they were more like brothers. He trusted Rick completely. Beyond the financial assistance, Frank had also supported his friend emotionally throughout the whole grieving process of his broken marriage.

Two years had gone by and Rick had recovered financially. It was now Frank who was going through a challenging time. He and his wife could not afford the new payment on their home because of an increase in their interest rate. To make matters worse, Frank's wife lost her job. They were on the brink of losing their home and Frank desperately needed to refinance with a larger down payment to modify his loan rate and monthly fee.

When Frank asked Rick if he could reimburse him the money, Rick said he would not be able to. He was starting a side business for which he needed to use all the money he had saved during the past year. Frank did not ask twice. He was stunned. After a few seconds of total shock, Frank left Rick's office without saying a word and went back to his home.

That night, while his wife was sound asleep, Frank was wide awake. He was devastated, shocked, and so disgusted by Rick's reaction that he felt nauseated. His perception of what Rick did to him was "indigestible," and he found it unacceptable. Frank spent every second dwelling on the situation, unable to sleep or eat for three days. He did not want to speak to anyone about it, not even his wife, and over the course of his constant thinking, he was unable to find a liberating solution of any kind. No matter how he looked at it, Frank could not "digest" the fact that Rick would not pay him back.

Frank and the fox have a lot in common: they both had a morsel too big to digest, only for the fox the morsel was real and for Frank the morsel was symbolic. Frank's conflict originated in the mind, while the fox's conflict originated in the stomach. Frank's "felt experience" will be interpreted metaphorically by his brain, which will respond as if a real morsel was stuck in Frank's stomach and needed to be broken down or passed through. The content of the mental conflict will be reduced to a metaphor, which simply indicates that there is a "morsel" in his stomach that is too big to be digested and processed. Frank's perception will consequently awaken and manifest one of the programs of adaptation related to digestion, i.e. stomach cancer.

When no solution is found by the mind, the brain transfers the conflict from the psychological sphere into the biological domain where a solution can be expressed. The brain will target the organ that corresponds exactly to the "felt experience." The question we might ask ourselves is: why is the cancer in Frank's stomach considered the ultimate solution by the brain versus letting Frank struggle with his mental battle? How is an illness such as cancer in any way profitable to a human being as a response to an emotional struggle? The answer becomes logical as soon as we understand the functioning of our nervous system.

SURVIVAL

The Autonomic Nervous System

The sympathetic nervous system is part of the autonomic nervous system. It permits the activation of neuronal and hormonal stress response, commonly known as the *fight-or-flight response*. When the nervous system recognizes the signals of a threatening environmental stress, the hypothalamus and pituitary gland will prepare the body's organs for action by informing the adrenal glands of the need to manage the fight-or-flight response. Subsequently, the release of adrenaline in the body will modify our physiology in order to provide us with great power to fend off or flee danger.

As human beings, we experience a certain amount of stress in our daily lives, whether it's arriving on time, paying our bills, dealing with work, maintaining a relationship, raising children, or driving in traffic. Fortunately, we are able to cope and adapt to most of our usual, momentary, and expected fears. We find solutions as we go through life and create ways to meet our vital needs. Most of our stresses are chronic, but not acute enough to threaten our survival. Considering we are able to create solutions relatively quickly, we are able to recover emotionally and, therefore, our bodies are allowed biological recuperation under the control of the parasympathetic nervous system.

The parasympathetic nervous system, also part of the autonomic nervous system, complements the sympathetic nervous system by regulating visceral organs and muscle contractions, thus permitting us to rest and digest after a phase of stress. We are under the control of the parasympathetic system every time we fully rest, sleep, and recover.

Unmanageable Stress

Unfortunately, sometimes our level of stress can trespass the threshold of what we can humanly bear, such as the death of a loved one, a divorce or separation, the loss of a job and security, or a betrayal. As described by Dr. Hamer, an event we did not anticipate that creates a highly acute, isolating shock (meaning an experience we cannot fully express) can trigger a peak state of stress.

We stay under the control of the sympathetic nervous system for as long as we perceive a situation as a threat. In case of danger, our body is ready to expend a maximum of energy so we can survive and prevail in battle or during escape. The longer we undertake such stress, the longer we will be subjected to an acceleration of our heart rate and a constriction of blood vessels of the digestive tract. Subsequently, suitable absorption of nutrients will be suppressed. The adrenal stress hormone will also constrict the blood vessels in our forebrain (the center of reasoning), thus preventing us from accessing an analytic thinking process [Takamatsu, et al., 2003; Arnsten and Goldman-Rakic 1998; Goldstein, et al., 1996]. This corroborates the fact that our brain is designed to automatically solicit our primal instincts in face of danger versus using an intellectual process.

Imagine you're on a camping trip in the mountains and having a wonderfully peaceful time when suddenly a bear appears in your path. Since the brain perceives the situation as dangerous, it will need to permit environmental information to quickly be used to inform a behavioral reaction. Your instinct might be to run away from the bear as fast as you can and to jump in a lake. If you started to "evaluate the situation" by trying to remember a strategy you learned on a television program, it might be to your disadvantage. Similarly, students who are frightened and paralyzed by academic tests frequently mark wrong answers because they cannot properly access the needed information. These students are also in a "fight or flight" mode. The higher the stress, the more we lose access to logic and evolved intelligence in order to maintain a state of instinctual alertness. The lower the stress, the more capable we are of finding intellectual solutions.

As long as a situation is perceived as dangerous, even if the conflict involves stress in our emotional life, i.e. a painful separation or the loss of a loved one, the brain will react and stay alert to the environment from a primal perspective, thus soliciting the sympathetic nervous system and the fight-or-flight response. If our conscious mind cannot find a way out of the problem and instead dwells on it day and night in order to resolve it, our stress will persist. As expected, during such a state there exists very limited access to realism and mental resources. While in a period of acute stress we will not be able to sleep and we will lose our appetite, lose weight, and feel cold.

We can easily foresee the consequences of not sleeping or eating during times of acute stress. After a certain amount of time we could die of exhaustion or inadvertence (lack of awareness), since our attention span is limited to looking for a solution to the conflict we are compulsively thinking about. We would definitely be at risk from environmental dangers, such as cars or buses, which replace the archaic dangers we were exposed to throughout our evolution.

Because the evolutionary process has molded human behavior, our neurological pathways have been selected to increase the survival of the individual. The human brain can only act on our biology and not the environment itself. Unlike our conscious mind, our subconscious makes choices moment-to-moment, accessing stored data, and is not concerned with the future. If a level of unmanageable stress is reached, our subconscious will gather the information provided by the conscious mind, such as environmental components perceived through our five senses, as well as the thoughts and feelings associated with the present conflict. This will trigger a neurological response, independent of the conscious mind, which aims to increase survival. A new program will be expressed biologically, matching perfectly the content of our "felt experience." A modification will immediately start in the targeted organ, metaphorically solving the conflict.

As soon as the conflict is expressed in the organ, the level of stress lowers to where it becomes manageable. The blood constriction in the forebrain is alleviated, thus permitting us to have access to more coherent reasoning in our thinking process. We can be more alert to the environment and therefore safer. We eat, sleep, and function better, subsequently prolonging our lives (from moment to moment).

Because our conflict is still mentally unresolved, part of the memory of the conflict will be hidden in the depth of our subconscious mind, eventually creating a so-called "blind spot" (obscuration of our memory), permitting us to lose awareness regarding our conflict in order to stop being confronted by the stress it triggers. Our stress level has now become compatible with life. Ultimately, our system is allowing us more moments of survival by expressing an illness in place of the extreme stress that could prompt death more rapidly. For instance, after Frank's mind manifested the solution in his body, i.e. the beginning of an illness in the digestive tract, a stomach tumor, his level of stress lowered and he had limited access to the painful memories related to his experience. He was then able to function in the world.

For as long as the solution to resolve our conflict has not been attained, the biological response (Dis-Ease) will be maintained. Fortunately, sometimes through a change of circumstances or a shift in perception, emotional conflicts can resolve naturally, even when an individual is unaware of their existence (which can explain many spontaneous recoveries).

What we call "disease" represents, in fact, the perfect solution to the individual's mental conflict, whether its origins are ancestral or personal. Our brain is still using an archaic mode of action to maintain our species. We are still subjected to archaic responses that have been used by living beings since the beginning of time in order to adapt to the pressure of the environment.

Today, we can understand certain diseases by observing the natural behaviors of non-human animals. Ethology is a science that studies the ecology and evolution of animal behaviors. Research findings in this field have led to the identification of the origin of certain diseases. Aristotle (384 -322 BC) was already making connections between biological dysfunctions in humans and certain characteristics he could observe in non-human animals. For instance, when a female partridge and her offspring come face to face with a hunter, the female will roll on herself to the left and right, similar to having a sudden uncontrollable outbreak. This behavior occupies the attention of the hunter, who is intent on capturing the bird, and allows the partridge's offspring to escape. According to French doctor and researcher Gerard Athias, the odd behavior of the partridge helps us understand the cause of epilepsy and how it is rooted in one's desire to momentarily divert attention. For example, a child might have a seizure for the first time when his parents are having a fight, therefore attracting attention and putting a stop to imminent violence in order to protect his mother.

Just like every animal on this planet, we experience distress that is related to survival. Even though our consciousness is more evolved than other species, we produce the same type of biological responses to stress as many of them do. Our perception is subjective, and the associations we make between events and their meanings are subconscious.

Evolution

From Unicellular Organisms to Human Kind

Over the course of evolution, living beings had to adapt to challenges presented by the environment. In the oceans, about six hundred million years ago, after the emergence of unicellular organisms like Eukaryotes, a succession of small, accumulated, biological modifications led to the development of reproductively isolated populations, each new generation being slightly different from the preceding one. The way living beings evolved is directly related to the law of "cause and effect." Mutations within individual organisms sometimes provided advantages under certain environmental conditions, or "stresses," and those organisms with these mutations increased in number faster than those without the mutations. Adaptation was necessary for lineages to survive in the ever-changing environment.

Most often, when our circumstances create unmanageable stress, our brain will implement an archaic solution that modifies our physiology. This modification in our body will occur according to recorded evolutionary programs, which can be identified by observing the behavior of animals.

The biologist Jean Baptiste Lamarck (1744-1829) stated that animal organs and behaviors can change according to the environment and the animal's survival needs. He also hypothesized that those characteristics can be transmitted from one generation to the next. For instance, he proposed that the neck of the giraffe becomes longer each generation due to the need to reach the upper leaves of the trees. Lamarck also stated that every living organism, including humans, has a propensity to reach a greater level of perfection.

Organisms, since the beginning of life on the planet, have continued to evolve in response to their environments. Disease, within the context of evolutionary history, may be redefined as a meaningful biological emergency program. Today all those programs remain part of our imprints. They can resurface according to the solution our brain needs to extrapolate from its evolutionary memory. We use our biology to adapt to what we perceive as insurmountable.

Biological lineages have gone through evolutionary change, developing new organs to meet adaptive needs. Among those changes is the development of four embryonic layers in the brain in synchronicity with the development of the needed organs in the body.

The *endoderm* layer, controlled by the archaic *brainstem,* is linked to *vital organs* and their related basic functions, such as breathing, eating, digesting, eliminating, and reproducing. Ancient aquatic living creatures needed to ensure vital needs such as the intake of oxygen and catching morsels of food. As our ancestors evolved, they left the aquatic domain and became terrestrial, thus prompting the development of a new brain layer.

At this time, the need arose for the protection of a stronger skin layer in order to cope with rough terrain and extremes in weather and temperature. The *old brain mesoderm* layer, controlled by the part of our brain called the *cerebellum,* is linked to enveloping organs and functions to protect against harsh environment and predatory attacks. Later in the evolutionary development of the human brain, the *new brain mesoderm* controlled by the *cerebral medulla* appeared, thus enabling movement and locomotion through the development of a muscular and skeletal system, permitting hunting strategies to expand.

As evolution continued, living creatures began to exist in social groups and form bonds with other individuals of the same species. Along with those bonds came the fear of losing safety and the need for stability of territory, thus encouraging the evolution of territory marking and maintenance systems.

The youngest of our four embryonic layers is called the *ectoderm* and is controlled by the *cerebral cortex*. This layer controls organs whose functions permit us to mark and fight for the preservation of the territory and includes organs related to more advanced and intellectualized needs. The ectoderm also commands organs that originated from the need to more accurately see, hear, and feel for the purpose of anticipating potential dangers.

Embryonic Layers

In most animals, *embryogenesis* starts as soon as fertilization of the egg occurs. In human beings, the four embryonic (germ) layers (endoderm, old and new mesoderm, and ectoderm) develop within the first twenty-one days of the embryonic life. In other words, a fetus at its earliest stage of development will undergo all the evolutionary stages of its phylogeny with a tremendously accelerated speed (from a single cell organism to a human being).

From those four stages of the brain development, we can deduce four families of Biological Conflicts:

The endoderm. The endoderm (inner germ layer), controlled by the brainstem, is the oldest layer that forms and commands *vital organs* such as the mouth, lower part of the esophagus, lungs, liver, pancreas, stomach, colon, kidney collecting tubule, prostate, and uterus.

The biological conflicts related to endodermal tissues are associated with the individual's vital needs, such as the ability to breathe, having enough to eat, or being able to process food. For instance, in a figurative sense, if a person is subjected to a "death-fright conflict" after being given a negative prognosis, the genes of his pulmonary alveoli might mutate, enabling a cell multiplication in the lung for the purpose of being able to get more oxygen and continue breathing. Other examples may include:

- A concern about lack of money and food can represent a conflict related to the fear of starvation. It is the role of liver cells, or hepatocytes, to maximize digestion. The proliferation of such cells, resulting in a tumor in the liver, expresses a subconscious need to make the most out of a small amount of food while subconsciously fearing famine.

- A profound tragedy, such as the loss of a child, might affect the mother's ovary by triggering a cell proliferation to achieve faster reproduction and metaphorically allow replacement of the deceased offspring.

The old brain mesoderm. The old brain mesoderm (part of the middle germ layer), controlled by the cerebellum, forms and commands organs linked to the *protection* of the organism, also described as *enveloping organs,* such as the corium skin, pleura, peritoneum, pericardium, and breast glands.

The biological conflicts related to the *old mesoderm* are connected to emotional stresses that concern attacks against one's integrity and can, as always with conflicts, be experienced literally and figuratively. For instance, an individual can be vulnerable to a verbal attack just as if real arrows were being shot at his heart. In this case, thickening of the pericardium (double walled sac that protects the heart) would safeguard the individual against further attacks, leading to pericardial mesothelioma, a rare cancer that develops in the membrane surrounding the heart. Other examples may include:

- A man might perceive lung surgery as an attack against his chest, and the pleura (two-layered membrane that protects the lung) would be the targeted organ to express such conflict. This could result in a mesothelioma of the pleura.

- When one's integrity is affected by a disagreeable physical contact, a feeling of being "stained" will emerge, which might affect the skin and trigger the development of a melanoma (cancer of the skin).

- A need to protect and nurture the offspring or partner could affect a woman's breast glands and trigger the proliferation of "milk producing cells" (breast cancer), which will allow the woman to symbolically "nurture" by providing more milk for the benefit of one of her loved ones.

The new brain mesoderm. The new brain mesoderm (part of the middle germ layer), controlled by the *cerebral medulla*, forms and commands organs related to *movement* such as bones, tendons, ligaments, connective tissue, muscles, most of the lymphatic system, blood vessels (with the exception of the coronary vessels), and the adrenal cortex.

The biological conflicts related to the *new mesoderm* are predominantly associated with self-depreciation, such as feeling insignificant in comparison with others. For instance, in an athletic environment, a gymnast specializing in "still rings" might feel devaluated after the arrival of a seemingly more talented teammate and will develop tendonitis in his arms as a result of such conflict. Other examples may include:

- A woman who feels her femininity has vanished and considers herself worthless as a sexual partner might suffer from a self-devaluation conflict that will affect her pubic bone with osteoporosis or even cancer, depending on the intensity of her "felt experience."
- Sometimes an individual can experience a state of powerlessness and defenselessness on a psychological level, thus leading to a reaction in the lymph nodes and perhaps the onset of lymphoma. The lymphatic system, which transports immune cells to and from the lymph nodes, figuratively represents our defense mechanisms. When one feels attacked, an ulceration within the lymphatic system permits a greater pathway for lymphocytes and monocytes to operate and "defend" the organism.

The new mesoderm is also linked to conflict related to "direction." A conflict of "having been thrown off course" or of "having gone in the wrong direction" in life, might lead to the decrease of adrenal function, which will elicit exhaustion, forcing the individual to stop pursuing the wrong path.

The ectoderm. The ectoderm (part of the outer germ layer), controlled by the *cerebral cortex*, forms and commands organs such as the epidermis, nasal and sinus membranes, inner ear, retina, bronchia, lining of the milk ducts, cervix, vagina, lining of the lower part of the rectum, lining of the bladder and the coronary vessels. The ectoderm is also linked to meaningful functional impairments such as diabetes and motor paralysis.

The biological conflicts of the ectoderm are related to territorial conflicts as well as sexual conflicts, existential conflicts, and motor conflicts. Some examples may include:

- An elderly man may have a difficult time "marking" his territory since his son and family have moved into his house and, for practical purposes, the man had to move his bed and sleep in the living room. To resolve his conflict, the old man will subconsciously trigger the ulceration of the tissue lining of his bladder. In this case, the biological meaning of the tissue loss is to allow the bladder to expand so that more urine can be contained and used to mark this man's territory, thus forcing the recognition of his position and boundaries.

- A woman might have to endure a job she despises, perhaps working in a factory where animals are being slaughtered. While she "resists" a repugnant situation, constant muscle tension in her body will require a greater glucose supply. Over time, her sugar levels will rise in the blood stream, thus leading to diabetes.

THE ONTOGENETIC SYSTEM OF TUMORS & CANCER EQUIVALENT DISEASES (According to Dr. Hamer)

TYPE OF EMBRYONIC LAYER	ENDODERM	OLD MESODERM	NEW MESODERM	ECTODERM
COMMAND RELAYS	BRAIN STEM	CEREBELLUM	CEREBRAL MEDULLA	CEREBRAL CORTEX
CORRESPONDING TYPES OF ORGANS & CONFLICTS	-Vital organs *Conflicts of the "Morsel" of oxygen or food (catching, digesting, assimilating, evacuating)* -Reproductive system *Conflicts of reproduction*	-Organs related to protection& integrity *Attack Conflicts* -Organs related to life preservation *Nest conflicts*	-Organs related to locomotion & circulatory organs *Conflicts of devaluation* -Some reproductive organs *Loss conflicts*	-Organs related to communication (five senses) *Conflicts of Separation* -Organs related to territory&boundaries *Territorial conflicts (Also motor conflicts & sexual/reproductive conflicts)*
EXAMPLES OF ORGANS IN CORROLATION WITH EVOLUTIONNARY STAGES	•Appendix •Bladder (submucosal) •Colon •Duodenum •Esophagus (lower) •Fallopian Tubes •Intestines •Kidney collecting tubule •Liver •Lung (Alveoli) •Mouth •Ovarian and Testicular teratoma* •Palate •Pancreas •Parathyroid gland •Parotid gland •Pharynx •Prostate Gland	•Breast (Milk gland) •Dermis •Meninges of the brain •Omentum •Pericardium of the heart •Peritoneum of the intestines •Pleura of the lungs •Shingles*	•Adrenal glands •Arterial blood vessels •Bladder sphincter •Blood vessels •Cartilage •Connective & fat tissue •Dentine •Kidney parenchyma •Lymph nodes •Muscles •Ovarian parenchyma •Rectum sphincter •Skeleton •Spleen •Tendons/Ligaments •Testicular parenchyma	•Alopecia* •Blader mucosa •Breast (intraductal) •Bronchi •Cervix •Coronary arteries •Cornea •Diabetes* •Epidermis •Esophagus (upper) •Glaucoma* •Hypoglycemia* •Larynx •Mouth (upper mucosa) •Multiple sclerosis* •Nervous system •Pancreatic ducts •Parotid Gland duct •Rectum (lower)

	FUNGI	MYCOBACTERIA	BACTERIA	VIRUSES
	• Rectum (Sigmoid) • Salivary gland • Stomach (exept small curvature) • Thyroid (Old) • Tonsils • Uterus			• Sinus mucosa • Stomach mucosa • Thyroid (new) • Urethral mucosa • Vagina • Vertigo*
CONFLICT ACTIVE PHASE	CELL MULTIPLICATION Mass formation	CELL MULTIPLICATION Mass formation	CELL REDUCTION Necrosis (tissue loss/holes)	CELL REDUCTION Ulceration (tissue loss) or loss of function (blocking)
CONFLICT RESOLUTION PHASE (Recovery)	CELL REDUCTION Necrosis / Ulceration	CELL REDUCTION Necrosis / Ulceration	CELL MULTIPLICATION	CELL MULTIPLICATION

ONTOGENETIC SYSTEM OF MICROBES

	FUNGI	MYCOBACTERIA	BACTERIA	VIRUSES
ACTIVE MICROBES DURING REPAIR PHASE (Infectious state)	Cell decomposition through caseous necrotization	Cell decomposition through caseous necrotization Ex : BK/Tuberculosis	Repair and restoration of ulcers	Repair and restoration of ulcers

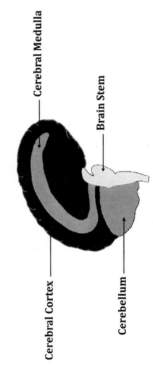

Cerebral Medulla

Brain Stem

Cerebral Cortex

Cerebellum

ILLNESS

The Role of Germs

Disease is nothing less than a useful biological change that permits adaptation during situations of danger. All the adaptation systems, such as tissue and organ modifications that developed over millions of years of evolution, are stored in our brain and in our genes. During a phase of high stress, when individuals are subjected to the action of the sympathetic nervous system, the function of organs can be modified. The functionality of an organ is enhanced or decreased by a cell proliferation, a cell meltdown, or specific hormonal variations to facilitate the resolution of the emotional conflict.

Up until now, Western medicine has been focusing on organs only and attributing their malfunctions to environmental toxicity, mechanical causes, viruses and bacterial "attacks," as well as considering infections as illnesses on their own. The events occurring after sustaining a skin laceration may illustrate the role microorganisms play in our basic biology.

Immediately after a laceration takes place, platelets stick together to create a scab and protect the region. Underneath the scab, new skin cells multiply with the help of germs, which optimize the reconstruction of a new layer of skin. Once the wound is repaired and a new layer is completed, the scab falls off. What is happening outside of our body is similar to what is happening inside. The body knows how to repair itself, and it seems bacteria have a specific role to play in our biology and are necessary for the restoration of our tissues.

While looking for the source of illness everywhere else, other than the individual's computer—the brain—the priority of Western medicine has been to "strengthen the immune system" by destroying germs. Microbes were the first form of life to develop on earth and have supported the development of plant and animal life throughout the course of evolution. These organisms operate as decomposers and expellers of foreign bodies within the biological system. They are present at all times in the human flora as well as in the cells. According to what Dr. Hamer refers to as "the ontogenetic system of microbes," germs do not proliferate unless repair is needed in the system, provided the necessary microbes are available. Interestingly, it was never considered that microbes might become purposely virulent in one's body according to precise organic needs and that the source of their flare-ups and occasional proliferation might actually have been initiated by the host system!

Pierre Bechamp, biologist and Professor of Pharmacology at the University of Montpellier, discovered microorganisms and demonstrated that germs are part of our system and constitute what he called "the terrain" in our biology. Unfortunately, Louis Pasteur's Germ Theory, which states that "germs invade our body from the outside world," has long been accepted as true. Pasteur not only plagiarized what Bechamp discovered six years earlier but also perverted the facts and influenced the foundation of Western medicine with distorted and inaccurate information. Pasteur actually admitted this act of plagiarism on his deathbed. A direct challenge to the Germ Theory took place when a man who wanted to prove the theory wrong deliberately drank a glass of water containing a substantial amount of *Vibrio cholerae*, a pathogen scientists assumed was responsible for acute intestinal infection. The man remained unaffected by the infectious agent. The scientists did not investigate this event further, and the experiment was disregarded [DiRita 2000].

Viruses, as well as bacteria, play an important role during the healing phase of certain diseases and behave according to the solicitation of our system. For instance, the fact that the flu virus will manifest itself every year within only a small percentage of individuals is not related to the strength of immune systems in the population, but rather the type of conflict a flu-exposed individual might be resolving. The flu virus optimizes the repair phase of the bronchial mucosa, which can be affected during the active phase of a small but intense human conflict, such as a dispute of territorial nature related to family or work. This type of conflict is common; that is why thousands of individuals are affected by the flu virus every year, providing the flu virus is present in their environment.

The Two Phases of Illness

When a conflict is resolved, the resulting illness develops in two phases: the *active phase* and the *healing phase.* The active phase starts at the time of the conflict shock (DHS) and continues as long as the individual has not resolved the emotional conflict related to the disease. Additionally, the size of a tumor will depend on the intensity and duration of the conflict.

The healing phase starts instantly at the moment the emotional conflict is resolved and permits the body to access the repair phase under the control of the parasympathetic system. The healing phase is elicited through two distinct pathways. The first pathway, called the "practical solution," is directly related to a change within the environment, which creates a context where the conflict no longer exists. For instance, in Julia's story, we could imagine that her husband returns after a few weeks with an explanation that is satisfying to her. Or, in Frank's case, the best friend apologizes and pays back the money he owed. In both situations, the environment itself provides the solution.

Is the problem resolved after the environment provides a solution? This solution may only be momentary since ultimately, if the original circumstances were to reoccur, the risk of a relapse would be significant.

The second pathway towards healing is through "the surpassing solution." When an individual is able to find (through a change of perception) a liberating solution to the distress, the healing phase can be set in motion. Ideally, this state of health will continue, no matter what fluctuations the environment brings in the future.

In order to access the surpassing solution, it is necessary for the individual to shift emotionally. This could involve ceasing to blame others for the conflict and starting to look at life as the unfolding of circumstances that permit growth. Easier said than done when our subconscious programs are running the show by influencing our perceptions and dictating our responses to the environment. Fortunately, certain therapies and their modalities (particularly NLP) permit us to gain new perceptions about our challenges as well as provide us with the necessary tools to take charge of our lives.

During the two phases of disease, biological modifications will take place according to the type of embryonic layer the emotional conflict solicits. It is important to note that organs and tissues controlled by the brainstem and cerebellum respond in opposite fashion compared to organs and tissues controlled by the cerebral medulla and the cerebral cortex.

Conflict active phase of illness. During the conflict active phase, also called "cold phase," the individual organism is under the control of the sympathetic nervous system. The higher the stress, the more an individual will undergo symptoms such as sleeplessness, lack of appetite, coldness, and elevated heart rate.

Organs controlled by the *endoderm* and *old mesoderm* germ layers will generate a cell multiplication during the active phase of a conflict. For example, during the active phase of a "nest-worry conflict," milk-producing cells will proliferate and create a tumor in a woman's breast glands (*old mesoderm).*

Organs controlled by the *new mesoderm* and *ectoderm* germ layers will undergo tissue loss during the active phase of a conflict (the ectoderm is also linked to the loss of function of certain organs). For example, during the active phase of a *separation conflict* an individual will develop skin ulcerations (epidermic ulcers) in order to reduce skin sensitivity. Figuratively, being desensitized and unable to "feel" permits an individual to bear the absence of another human being (such as a family a member), or any other absent element, and to sustain the distress related to separation. In other words, this loss of sensitivity represents a temporary memory lapse. For instance, the microscopic ulcerations (cell decrease) that precede the appearance of eczema won't be detected during the active phase of such conflict.

Healing phase of illness. Growths and tumors controlled by the *endo-derm* and *old mesoderm* germ layers (which develop during the active cold phase) are degraded with the help of fungi or bacteria during the healing, or warm, phase of the conflict. For example, during the healing phase of a "nest-worry conflict," a special program will be activated in order to decompose the tumor of the breast gland with the help of Tuberculosis bacteria.

Tissue loss, which occurs in organs controlled by the *new mesoderm* and *ectoderm* germ layers during the active phase, will be replenished with the proliferation of new cells and the intervention of bacteria and viruses (if available) during the healing phase. For example, during the resolution phase of a "separation conflict" an individual will experience eczema, which corresponds to the skin restoration phase through ulcer replenishment. Such a condition becomes chronic only when a periodic relapse of the conflict of separation occurs.

What Dr. Hamer names *conflictolysis* corresponds to the turning point between the conflict active phase and the healing phase. Just like the DHS (representing the dramatic shock), the healing phase starts simultaneously at three levels: the psyche, the brain, and the organ. As soon as the conflict is resolved in the psychological sphere (in one's mind), the individual feels a great emotional relief and the healing phase (*warm phase*) begins. When the healing phase begins, the autonomic nervous system reverts to the control of the parasympathetic system, thus permitting the individual to rest, regain appetite, and recuperate. Symptoms such as fever, swelling, inflammation, infection, pain, and headaches can occur, making this natural healing process difficult to bear and sometimes dangerous.

According to Dr. Hamer, an episode called the *Epileptoid Crisis* occurs simultaneously on all three levels (psyche, brain, organ) during the height of the healing phase. It is a brief "stress relapse" that permits the flushing out of the edema surrounding the "command relay" of the brain after repair has been initiated in both areas (the brain and the organ). The consequent part of the healing phase follows its course with the formation of scar tissue.

Illness is a reversible process, but the healing phase is rarely asymptomatic. Because of a lack of information, most individuals disregard the meaning of its course and interrupt it instead of gently monitoring some of its unpleasant symptoms, such as fatigue, pain, fever, inflammation, infection, and headache. According to Dr. Hamer, we often attempt to abruptly eliminate such signs through the use of medication, which oftentimes interferes with the natural repair of the body.

On the other hand, the natural healing phase of certain conflicts can be dangerous, and individuals may benefit from the advanced techniques of Western medicine. For example, where a conflict of territorial loss is concerned, the heart will be affected during the healing phase. In such case, a better understanding about the two phases of illness might permit the anticipation and even prevention of heart failure.

Healing phase of a territorial loss conflict. There are three main types of territorial conflicts: the conflict related to "territorial loss" will affect the heart, the conflict linked to "marking territory" will affect the bladder or rectum, and the "human conflict related to aerial territory" (disputes) will affect the bronchi. The origin of heart disease can be understood through the observation of animal combat over territory.

Every year during the mating period for bull elk, the dominant bull elk is challenged by young rivals for the right to mate. If the dominant bull wins the fight, it will remain the dominant elk in his population and will be the only male allowed to mate with the females of his herd, ensuring his genetic contribution to the next generation. During such extreme fighting with the challenging elk, intense strength (muscle power) is needed during a short period of time. Throughout the combat, the inner lining of the coronary arteries will ulcerate, increasing their diameter, thus allowing for a greater quantity of blood and oxygen to be pumped and distributed to the entire body.

This biological solution increases the chances for each male elk to win the fight related to territory. It is by far more vital for the dominant bull elk to keep his position and triumph over his rival, because he has everything to lose compared to the young buck that never owned territory and harems. In this case, the dominant bull elk will keep fighting until complete exhaustion, even in cases when he is losing the battle.

At the end of combat, a new biological response will take place so that the lining of the coronary arteries (intima) can be repaired. The restoration of the intima will involve an increase of cholesterol, which acts to replenish the micro-ulcerations of the coronaries during the healing phase. Even though the male bull elk does not intake excess cholesterol, its arteries can still carry an overload of cholesterol. However, the reason dominant bull elks die of heart failure is not directly related to the blockages cholesterol plaques might create.

According to Western medicine, heart attacks are related to blockages in the arteries impairing blood supply and preventing enough oxygen from getting to the heart. Dr. Hamer advocates that heart failures are directly related to the conflict of territorial loss and the variations the brain is subjected to during the healing phase of such conflict.

Remember that when the healing phase starts, the organ and its brain relay are undergoing repair simultaneously with the appearance of an edema (interstitial fluid). The size of the edema encompassing the brain relay related to the coronaries (cortex) can create danger. Its size is proportional to the duration of the territorial distress and can sometimes become relatively large. The process of elimination of such edema (which occurs in the middle of the repair phase— epileptoid crisis) will create a momentary disturbance that will affect surrounding regions of the brain, thus stimulating relays that are connected to the functioning of the heart. One neurological relay in particular might be triggered, thus provoking bradycardia (heart slowness) or even cardiac arrest. The origin of heart failure hides behind the mechanisms, which take place during the healing phase of a territorial conflict. We may wonder: if nature is so clever, why does the so-called "healing phase" lead to death after an intense territorial conflict? Again, the answer lies within the survival archetypes of the species.

For instance, it is in the best interest of the species that the bull elk does not return to his herd after he loses his fight, since it would disturb the young bucks that would be fighting instead of mating. Such interference would lower the number of offspring being conceived. Female elk have a short estrus cycle of only a couple of days where successful mating can occur. In order to insure the next generation, mating needs to happen timely and in alignment with the seasons, so the calves will then benefit from the camouflage the forest can provide and have a better chance to avoid being seen by predators. After the dominant elk loses, his death through a massive heart attack becomes the perfect solution for the propagation of the species.

Nature provides two types of survival programs. One program is that of personal survival, giving both participants a chance to win by enlarging the diameter of their coronary arteries thus giving them more strength to fight. The other program is related to the survival of the herd, when after the fight, the ideal solution for the species prevails and leads the older bull elk to die of a heart failure.

If the young buck is losing, it does not insist on fighting relentlessly and will stop before exhausting itself. Although its need for territory is instinctual, it is not as strong as for the dominant bull elk, which already has the habit of owning his territory and females. When recuperating after the fight, the healing phase for the young buck will be smooth, thus allowing its survival. The young elk will fight again the following year to win its territory. As years go by and the dominant elk becomes older and weaker, the chances for the young buck to become dominant will progressively increase.

When a human loses his or her territory, he or she will trigger the same biological program experienced by the bull elk, and his or her coronary arteries will ulcerate for as long as the fight for territory is sustained, whether real or figurative. For instance, when a man loses an essential component of his environment such as his job, house, wife, or group of friends, he might "fight" to get his position back. This will trigger ulcerations for more blood flow in his coronary arteries while he is fighting to get back what belonged to him.

As explained earlier, when an issue perceived as territorial loss goes on for too long, the amplitude of the healing phase can be massive and can lead to heart failure. A heart attack is related to the conflict of territorial loss and is prompted during the repair phase of the coronaries brain relay. This can explain why people who exercise and lead a healthy life can suddenly have a heart attack (if they have intense stress related to territory).

It's not unusual for a man to have a heart attack a few months after retiring from his job. This is because he has lost his "territory," perhaps to a younger worker. Sometimes a football player can experience a massive heart attack during a game as he fights for his team to win. Also, we can observe more heart disease in women as they have masculine social positions in the world, strong roles to play in their community, more and more rights, and therefore territory they can lose. Again, these phenomena are related to our perceptions, which is why not every individual who loses a job, spouse, or house will experience a territorial loss in their psyche and trigger a heart problem.

Just like the heart, other organs controlled (or partially controlled) by the ectoderm such as the rectum, bladder, cervix, or esophagus can also manifest symptoms that can be unpleasant and distressing during the reparation phase. It is often through symptoms such as bleeding that illness is discovered and perceived as aggressive, which can be frightening.

Healing phase of a rectal cancer. Consider the example of a man who is undergoing rectal swelling and bleeding. Three months prior to these symptoms, the man had been fired from his job without an explanation and was shocked at how his boss treated him after twenty years of being an excellent employee. This conflict in his psyche led him to trigger a DHS (conflict shock). He felt as if he did not know where to belong after years of having the same position in the company. In other words he could not "mark his territory" any longer.

During the active phase of the conflict, the rectum (ectodermic layer in this case) will be subjected to a painless ulcerative widening that figuratively allows more room for defecation. This phenomenon figuratively permits an individual to reinforce the "marking" of his territorial position according to archaic programs (in nature, some mammals use scent-marking to signal the limit of their territories by defecation).

One day the same man runs into his former boss at the supermarket and finally has a conversation where he can express his feelings. At the same time, the boss has an opportunity to apologize and explain his situation. The man then understands it was not at all personal but a necessity for the company to lay off a couple of employees in order to survive and that his position had not been replaced. The boss even promises to rehire him if the situation improves. Symbolically, the man can still own his position after this conversation with his former boss.

Immediately following this conversation, the man resolves his emotional distress and subconsciously lets go of the conflict. There is no reason for the illness to continue and the ulcerations in the rectum are no longer necessary. The brain then switches its program to the healing phase, permitting the organism to recuperate under the control of the parasympathetic system. The swelling of the rectal mucosa during the healing phase corresponds to the restoration phase of the ulcerated tissue and thin blood will be present in the stool. The man believes he has hemorrhoids and goes to see his doctor. According to Dr. Hamer, the man might be diagnosed with rectal cancer as he is actually undergoing symptoms of the healing phase of the disease.

If we validate the two phases of an illness, the various types of symptoms we are subjected to during the course of a disease can finally be explained and anticipated. Once an individual resolves an emotional conflict, the biological modification that momentarily took place during the conflict needs to be reversed. In other words, the organs need to be restored to their original healthy state. For this to happen, growths and tumors need to be encased or decomposed, while ulcerations need to be repaired and replenished with new cells. During the healing phase of an illness, microorganisms such as fungi, microbes, bacteria, and viruses will be used by the system as optimizers to rehabilitate the proper functioning of the organs. As a result, infection, fever, and inflammation will arise as secondary symptoms as soon as the healing phase begins.

A healing phase can be interrupted if there is a recurrence of a high stress state. The brain will halt the healing phase in favor of dealing with the new stress and mobilize energy to "fend or flee" danger, eventually re-triggering a DHS. For instance, a woman might be in a healing phase of intraductal cancer (breast cancer of the milk ducts) because she has resolved a separation conflict (related to the nest) with her husband whom she is no longer divorcing. When her doctor tells her that her prognosis is bad, she has an extreme fear of dying. Ultimately, she will once again undergo a high level of stress, which could trigger a secondary cancer in the lung. It is necessary, therefore, to look at the connection between secondary stresses and secondary tumors and to re-evaluate their origin.

Possible Origin of Metastases

According to Western medicine, cancer cells break away from primary tumors, enter the lymphatic system, and circulate through the bloodstream, subsequently affecting other organs and their tissues, where they will start proliferating. Modern medicine has never satisfactorily explained why the metastases of most cancers seem to be "organized" and why they generally follow the same path according to the origin of the primary cancer. For instance, breast cancer is often found in the liver, bones, and lung. Colon cancer may also appear in the liver, while prostate cancer will frequently manifest exclusively in the bone as a secondary location.

If it is true that cancer cells migrate erratically, why would these cells so often systematically follow the same course for the same type of cancer? Could it be possible that the course a cancer will take is determined by a logical combination of conflicts, which often create the same domino effect, resulting in the same systematic layout of secondary locations?

With all due respect to Western medicine, oncologists are not able to precisely define the cause of cancer nor the mechanism behind secondary locations of most cancers. Often times, medical prognoses are solely based on statistics. Consequently, in cases where there is unexpected cell activity, there are even fewer answers. For instance, finding a metastasis of lung cancer in the spleen is considered rare and out of the norm.

According to Dr. Hamer, the spread of cancer to secondary locations does not manifest in the way described by Western medicine, i.e. through blood and lymphatic circulation. Dr. Hamer describes how several conflicts can manifest in conjunction with one another, as the perception related to one dramatic experience might awaken multidimensional feelings. In that case, during the occurrence of a dramatic experience, several areas of the brain can be impacted at the same time, resulting in multiple "conflict shocks" and the manifestation of various simultaneous diseases.

For instance, a woman goes through a divorce and finds out her husband is planning on leaving her penniless with absolutely no consideration for her needs. She perceives her husband's behavior toward her as vile and disgusting, thus triggering colon cancer. At the same time she is worried that she might be unable to sustain and feed herself and her children. This perception may elicit a *starvation conflict* and lead to the manifestation of liver cancer. Her feeling of *worthlessness* could trigger bone cancer, since she feels the distress of a global self-devaluation. In that case, the bone cancer would produce a skeletal manifestation such as osteolysis (cell decrease), symbolically matching the woman's perception of being *nothing* and her subconscious intent to disintegrate.

The stress accompanying a cancer diagnosis and often its negative prognosis may trigger biologic responses that are relevant to subsequent disease outcomes [Andersen, B.L., et al., Psychologic Intervention Improves Survival for Breast Cancer Patients: A Randomized Clinical Trial. *Cancer,* 2008. 113: p. 3450-3458].

A negative prognosis can generate a secondary conflict in one's psyche due to the triggering of the fear of death. For example, the impact of frightening predictions could produce an unmanageable "death-fright-conflict," leading an individual to lung cancer (since alveoli cells process oxygen) as a cancer concomitant to the primary one.

Although all traumas do not always seem to provoke an illness or symptom, the traumas and their accompanying solutions (whether behavioral or biological) are memorized, consequently becoming subconscious imprints. Nothing is ever forgotten emotionally; therefore, past traumas are often precursor programs to illnesses.

Some individuals who have been close to death recall seeing their entire life passing in front of their eyes, just like an accelerated film replaying all their experiences. In those few seconds, since death is imminent, the subconscious mind rapidly searches for a solution, trying to access a stored program that exists in some part of that person's life and that could be re-activated to permit survival. The primary function of our brain is to keep us alive, and that is why it will keep in "storage" every biological solution and useful behavioral strategy, whether archaic, ancestral, parental, or personal, and either pleasant or unpleasant.

The Programming and Triggering Factors of Illness

There are three principal ways a person can trigger a disease through the impact of individual experiences. These disease triggers will be described using examples of some dramatic cases.

First Possibility: The programming of an illness and its trigger are simultaneous. This disease trigger involves a specific type of stress that occurs for the very first time in a person's life. There is no previous imprint of the same nature.

Caroline is experiencing emotional distress at the age of fifty-nine related to her grandchild's accidental death at the playground. This stress triggers breast cancer. It is the first time in her life that Caroline has experienced a "nest-worry conflict." Her brain is imprinting a stress and is triggering an illness simultaneously, similar to the case of Dr. Hamer, who never seemed to have experienced a dramatic and profound loss before the death of his son Dirk. In his case as well as Caroline's, the first mental impact or conflict prompted the illness.

Second possibility: The programming of an illness and its trigger are at a distance in time. At the age of twenty-six, Sandy loses her two-year-old daughter in a car accident and is experiencing a "profound loss conflict," which will start affecting one of her ovaries (a cell proliferation permits metaphorically to achieve faster reproduction to replace the deceased offspring). She gets pregnant three weeks after the loss of her child. Sandy believes in reincarnation and attributes her new pregnancy to the return of her daughter. Her perception permits her to find a satisfying solution to her stress and to resolve her profound emotional loss conflict. The start of the biological modification in the ovary will remain unnoticed, although an imprint of the emotional impact of profound loss and all it entails will remain, establishing a "first program," or first emotional imprint, in her subconscious mind.

When Sandy's second daughter is diagnosed with leukemia at age five, Sandy will re-experience a "profound loss conflict" as she anticipates the death of this child. Since her doctor does not give her the certainty that her daughter is going to live, Sandy stays in a state of unmanageable stress for too long. Her subconscious mind will automatically ensure survival on its own terms by awakening the program she imprinted five years earlier (when she lost her first child), which is of the same nature as the conflict she has about losing her second child. This will lead to ovarian cancer.

Sometimes several stresses of the same nature can accumulate during one's lifetime before the triggering moment of a disease.

Third possibility: A big stress awakens other stresses that are not correlated in terms of "meaning" and "conflict content." At the age of fifty-one, Jeffrey, who lives alone, loses his house to a fire and shortly after, his vision is severely impaired by an acute eye inflammation. We could at first anticipate that his eye problem is related to the fact that he will never "see" his house again, or the objects he was attached to that burned in the fire. Since he saw his house burn, we might also be inclined to think his eye problem occurred because subconsciously he didn't want to experience seeing his house being destroyed in front of his eyes. But this is not the case. In fact, when his stress level was at a peak, while watching the dramatic event unfold, Jeffrey's subconscious brain was actively searching for a stored solution that would lower his high level of stress. Since there were no stored memories that immediately resonated with this unexpected, distressing experience, Jeffrey's brain awakened a response which corresponded to another stress of similar intensity but different in its content.

When he was seven years old, instead of giving him his usual cleaning eye drops, his mother mistakenly gave him a different medication that belonged to his dad. Although this medication did not burn young Jeffrey's eyes, it created temporary blindness, resulting in a state of fear and a peak level of stress. This event was followed by a terrible eye inflammation, restoring the damage caused by the medication. Years later, when his house burned down, Jeffrey's subconscious mind awakened the biological response associated with the stressful experience forty-four years prior (eye inflammation). The brain, operating just like a computer's search engine, connected together two events that were totally different in terms of "meaning" but equivalent in terms of stress and intensity. A big stress can awaken any old stress and its corresponding biological response.

The phenomena of the programming and triggering of illness has been extensively described by Dr. Claude Sabbah (Total Biology of the Living Beings), whose remarkable analysis of disease triggers helps us understand the depth of our biological makeup.

Discovery Upon Discovery

Total Biology

In the early 90's, Dr. Sabbah expanded on the extraordinary findings of the New Medicine of Dr. Hamer by creating the concept of *The Total Biology of the Living Beings*. This concept represents forty years of Dr. Sabbah's personal research, analysis, and integration of Western medicine, the New Medicine of Dr. Hamer, the Bio-memorized Cellular Cycles and Project-Purpose of Dr. Marc Frechet, the Psycho-genealogy of Anne Ancelin Schützenberger, and various other modalities. He was the first to combine all the above concepts, thus creating an unprecedented methodology to help individuals resolve their subconscious stress.

Dr. Sabbah was able to synthesize information from various disciplines with the intention of furthering the understanding of the origin of emotional conflicts and disease. During this period, he wrote a reference book called *The Biological Decoding*, in which he ingeniously describes the biology of living beings, comparing the three domains: plant, animal, and human. Through his research, Dr. Sabbah was able to clearly understand the archetypes governing life and created the first practical therapeutic approach to resolve conflicts leading to illness.

The rapid expansion of Dr. Sabbah's Total Biology® concept permitted the general public to have access to German New Medicine through seminars. This concept was introduced in the early 90's, earlier than expected by Dr. Hamer, who was far from being recognized and accepted by the medical establishment. During the time Dr. Sabbah studied New Medicine (which became known as German New Medicine®) with Dr. Hamer, the knowledge of the link between emotional conflicts and disease was mainly intended for health professionals.

Since 1997, the concept of Total Biology® has become extensively propagated in Europe and North America due to the fact that early students of Dr. Sabbah, such as Gerard Athias, Bertrand Lemieux, and Christian Fleche, among others, reproduced, taught, and sometimes expanded on this theory of understanding the root of illness. Even though Total Biology® grew in recognition, the fact still remains that German New Medicine® was the foundation and the predecessor of many subsequent ideologies.

Dr. Sabbah developed brilliant metaphors that precisely connect disease to their specific emotional source. This methodology permits messages and their healing solutions to break through the barrier of one's subconscious, resulting in immediate insight about the conflict. Numerous individuals were able to find solutions to their health conditions while attending Sabbah's seminars. Among the metaphors developed by Dr. Sabbah is the extraordinary story of "Joey the Hunter," a caveman whose intense psychological conflict leads him to illness.

The Story of Joey (by Dr. Claude Sabbah)

Prehistoric humans used caves as shelter and protection from predators and environmental elements. In the case of Joey, he and his fellow hunters have to wade through a river running through a valley in order to reach a forest where prey is abundant. Unfortunately, the river is infested with a multitude of deadly, venomous snakes and, because the hunters are shoulder-deep in water, they risk getting bitten by these snakes.

Joey has a terrible fear, intensified every time he has to cross the river, since he has a memory of his grandfather dying from a snakebite twenty-five years prior, and both his father and brother succumbing to the same fate a few years later. Sadly, the most recent victim was Joey's best friend, who also died of a snakebite.

Considering the fate of the men in his family and his best friend, each time Joey has to go hunting, his heart rate is elevated, he breaks into a cold sweat, and he has to deploy a superhuman effort in order to follow his companions and cross the river. The deeper he goes into the water, the higher his stress level climbs, and his brain records the metaphor *descent equals danger*. Halfway crossing the river, his stress level peaks. When the *ascent* begins, Joey's fear starts to diminish, but instead of being relieved, a strong emotional state of self-devaluation overwhelms him, which is also recorded by his brain. Joey compares himself to his courageous fellow hunters and sees himself as a coward. He is now experiencing a double conflict, one connected with *movement* (in this case a *vertical movement* when he goes down into the river), and the other with *self-devaluation* (as he progressively gets out of the river and feels like a coward). Joey endures the conflict of "self-devaluation in a vertical movement" night and day as he constantly anticipates the next hunting trip. He needs an immediate solution, as he is continuously overstressed and could die from exhaustion (due to lack of sleep and loss of appetite) or the danger related to inadvertence (being distracted by his conflict and losing awareness of environmental dangers).

Joey needs to settle this conflict in his mind in order to resolve the situation. For instance, he could avoid crossing the snake-infested river by creating a bridge or a raft. Even though the snakes still exist, they would no longer pose a threat to Joey if he were to create a solution to surpass the problem. He could also decide to kill all the snakes one by one with a spear, no matter how long it would take him, thus eliminating the source of his issue in a practical way. In any of these cases, the conflict would be resolved and Joey's stress could be eliminated for good. There are always several solutions to a conflict, but if no satisfying solution is found by the individual, whether practical or one that surpasses the problem, the subconscious mind, whose purpose it is to prolong survival, will have to come up with an alternate solution.

Joey's brain cannot fix the environment. It can only act within the constraints of Joey's biology and send specific orders to manifest a change at a cellular level, such as cellular growth, tissue loss, or a loss of a function, in perfect accordance with Joey's type of conflict. In this case, the ultimate solution will be to *block a function* by triggering a paralysis so that Joey does not have to move anymore. The brain will send a special program in order to stop the production of myelin, which plays an essential role in the proper functioning of the nervous system. Myelin protects and insulates neurons. It also permits the quick and accurate transmission of electrical current data down the body of the nerve, thus enabling locomotion. In Joey's case, demyelization will occur, resulting in the disease we call Multiple Sclerosis (MS). MS will gradually permit him to stop moving. He will never again have to deal with the snakes and endure the stress of crossing the river. Joey will then be able to stay in the cave and, as a member of his tribe, settle into his new role of surveying the campfire, helping the females watch after their children, or guarding the cave. The other hunters will understand his misfortune, and Joey will not have to compare himself to them any longer and suffer the humiliation of feeling less than a man every time the rest of the tribe goes hunting. Since Joey cannot move, his conflict of self-devaluation associated to movement will somehow still be present but now transformed into a mild form of the conflict, in which the level of stress will be drastically diminished and therefore more viable.

With this story, Dr. Sabbah gives us a profound understanding of the idiosyncrasies accompanying the triggering of illness, making us realize that, although it might seem evident from our point of view that Joey should be able to find one of dozens of solutions available to him, it does not mean he will be able to manifest and be satisfied by any of them.

Similarly, when we look at others, we find ourselves observing their issues while feeling we would know exactly what to do in their circumstances. Most often, during an emotional crisis, the only viable solution is the one that is preferred by the conflicted individual. A woman having a partner conflict because her husband left her for another woman will not be satisfied unless her husband comes back to her. Instead, an alternate solution might be that she could choose to move on and create a new life for herself, perhaps with one of the millions of men still available on the planet. The man who loses his job to a younger man and perceives it as a territorial loss will want his old job back versus looking for a new one, deciding to start his own business, or seeing this time as an opportunity to take a sabbatical.

When one's reaction to an event seems out of proportion or irrational, it simply means an earlier painful memory, stored in the subconscious brain, is emerging. The root of our distress may certainly be found within our childhood, but nonetheless, it seems a whole chain of events and memories have already been assembled for us to undertake, surprisingly enough, even prior to the moment of our birth.

What Is Influencing
Our Destiny?

———

The Project-Purpose

The discoveries of the French clinical psychologist Marc Frechet, who died in 1997, enlightened us about the impact parents have on their offspring during gestation by what he called the "Project-Purpose." As human beings, we carry within our subconscious minds the memories of all the stages living beings endured throughout the course of evolution, thus enabling us to progress and subsist on the planet. Since the beginning of life, programs have been passed on from brain to brain, particularly from parents to offspring, in order to preserve the learning acquired during each experience where survival was at stake.

An experiment with earthworms is a perfect illustration of the impact an emotional distress can have on the next generation. In this experiment, an earthworm was being poked with a needle every time its container was subjected to direct sunlight. So, every time the worm was exposed to light, it felt pain and therefore associated light with danger. In an effort to save its life, the earthworm sought a place in the shadows, hiding in the corner of the container, seeking to end the pain. The worm associated light with pain, and the solution to survive this stress was to search for darkness. As a consequence of this emotional distress, the worm's offspring, as early as birth, repeated the same behavior of straying from light and finding refuge in the shadows, even though the offspring were never poked. The psychological conflict of the parent becomes "bio-logical" in the progeny. The information is passed on from brain to brain in order to save the species the time of relearning the strategy necessary for survival.

As human beings, we will express throughout our lifespan the solution or purpose we were meant to fulfill, according to the subconscious plan of one or both of our parents. For instance, if a pregnant woman feels a strong desire to divorce her husband but cannot fulfill her *project* because of the financial difficulties she would have to face (without the security offered by her husband's job), her unborn daughter might be predisposed to a certain path. The daughter would most likely be programmed to express the *winning solution* and liberate her mother's struggle later in her life by becoming financially independent and divorcing her own spouse. In this case, the daughter was subconsciously programmed to attract the *ideal* partner (a partner she would wind up divorcing) in order to express the *solution* connected to the *project* of her mother, i.e. finding financial independence and ending an unfulfilling marriage.

We will also be predisposed to recreating the *climate* that permeated the life of our parents during the time between our conception and the age of a least one year old. For example, the maternal climates of poverty and loneliness or abundance and joy could produce very different progeny. Interestingly, it has been observed by Dr. Gerard Athias, specialist in the field of Total Biology®, and confirmed by Gilbert Renaud, PhD (Recall Healing®), that even emotional stresses endured by the parents up to nine months before the conception of their child might also influence the future of the offspring. These subconscious imprints are often the origins of certain diseases.

A study conducted by the University of Copenhagen showed that people who were adopted at birth actually had a cancer risk similar to that of their adoptive parents, rather than that of the birth parents who gave them their genes. [Sorensen, T.I.A., et al., Genetic and environmental influences on premature death in adult adoptees. *New England Journal of Medicine*, 1988. 318: p. 727-32] This study reinforces the idea that the predisposition to certain disease is related to the transfer of subconscious emotional distress rather than genetic coding.

What we might consciously want to change in our lives does not stop our subconscious mind from completing its intrinsic programs of survival, consequently influencing our future and destiny. Since all of us are subjected to biological laws, we are not victims of our parents, but rather the recipients of information that will be processed and used according to the logic of our archaic brain. It is essential to remember that our parents cannot be held guilty for the programs they transmitted to us before, during, or after gestation, since they had no awareness of these imprints.

The moment of birth is unique and represents the first traumatic experience in life. After nine months of experiencing the safety of the uterus, an infant is suddenly exposed to the world. Elements surrounding the first moments of life outside of the womb will be deeply imprinted. The fears of the parents, their state of mind, their wants and needs will be embedded within the blueprint of a newborn.

A mother might hope for her child not to be born before her husband returns from a business trip so that he may witness the birth. Her emotional stress is related to timing of the birth and wanting to slow down a natural process that is imminent. Such distress around the moment of birth might affect the offspring in such fashion that it might program a behavior of always arriving late in life, subconsciously expressing loyalty to the survival need of the mother.

Our subconscious mind stores a considerable amount of additional memories besides our archaic biological codes of behavior. Everything that happens to us while we are alive, good or bad, is considered by our brain to be a strategy that allows the extension of our lives. For that purpose only, even negative shocking events such as accidents and illnesses have a tendency to reoccur in cyclical motions during our lifetime.

The Bio-Memorized Cellular Cycles

During his research, Marc Frechet uncovered the existence of Bio-Memorized Cellular Cycles and empirically demonstrated that events have a tendency to reappear in our lives in accordance with emotional impacts, which are memorized in the holographic system of our brain. The duration of a cycle is determined according to the age an individual becomes autonomous and capable of providing for oneself. This specific moment of independence is considered to be a recurrence of "birth" by the brain.

When we are born, we move away from the security of the womb. Similarly, when we become autonomous, we move away from the security of home and metaphorically "go out in the world." For example, a young woman who starts her first job at the age of 19 years and 3 months, rents her own apartment, and is in all respects completely independent from that time on, will have cycles of 19 years and 3 months. Her subconscious mind might attract circumstances to replay significant events from the "recorded tape" (events imprinted by the brain during the first cycle, from the time of birth until the age of 19 years and 3 months).

For example, if she was in a car accident with her parents at the age of 4, she might again have a car accident at 23 years and 3 months (19 years and 3 months + 4 years). If she had surgery at 10 years old, she might have another surgery at 29 years and 3 month old (19 years old and 3 months +10). If at 12 years old she received an award as the best student in her class, she might re-live a similar experience at 31 years and 3 months old (19 years old and 3 months + 12) when given an award for best sales person of the year by her company.

Illustration of Bio-Memorized Cellular Cycles

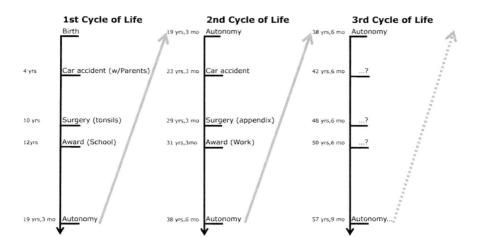

This amazing discovery of cyclical recurrence of life events, which has been verified by hundreds of therapists and their clients, permits us to understand that such repetitions in our lives are not due to hazard but rather a "co-incidence" of events related to certain dates and our cellular memory. Once we become aware of such cycles, it is possible to free ourselves from certain repetitions of unwanted events while still preserving positive reiterations. Beyond the influence of our life experiences during our time on earth and our time in the womb, there is also the influence of programs passed on from previous generations.

Transgenerational Transmission

Since childhood, Natalie, a young woman in her late twenties whom I met in 2005, possessed a constant fear of having an incurable illness and that one of her parents would die early. That constant fear fueled a feeling of heavy, seemingly incurable sadness. However, while investigating the life of her ancestors, she discovered that her despair might be directly related to the grief her grandmother experienced when she lost her five-year-old daughter (Natalie's aunt) to leukemia. Natalie's grandmother had struggled with the fact that she could not save her daughter from an incurable illness and was thus forced to watch her die at such an early age. Interestingly enough, Natalie went on to graduate with a PhD in Biology and chose to specialize in cancer research, subconsciously attempting to find a solution to her grandmother's distress by becoming an expert in the field of cancer.

Anne Ancelin Schützenberger, a psychologist, teacher and researcher at the University of Nice in France, is a renowned specialist in Transgenerational Therapy. In her book (*The Ancestor Syndrome: Transgenerational Psychotherapy and the Hidden Links in the Family Tree*, 1993), she describes how programs are passed on from one generation to the next and how our lives often reflect circumstances, traumas, and dates of events belonging to antecedent members of our clan. It appears we are not as free as we think and often express an invisible loyalty to our ancestors. What we call coincidences, such as the repetition of deaths at a certain age, separations, divorces, births, illnesses, and professional failures, are often related to unresolved stresses that reappear in our lives and will reappear in the lives of subsequent generations in order to be addressed and liberated. Freud described a similar phenomenon as "the return of elements that should have been surmounted a long time ago by our ancestors" ("Das Unheimlich," 1919) when he interpreted the repetitive nightmares of descendants of war survivors and the horrors they endured.

Throughout the course of our lives, we oftentimes express behavioral or biological solutions that permit us to resolve the stress of a parent or ancestor. It is interesting to note that our ancestors' reality, and most often their experienced suffering, is related to a belief system belonging to an ancient time. For instance, for the sake of family honor, a mother and daughter might have kept forever the secret of the daughter's illegitimate pregnancy by giving the child up for adoption. Such secrets, often perceived by the child and its mother as a stress related to abandonment, might predispose a member of the next generation to being overweight, since metaphorically the "bigger" we are if "abandoned in nature" the more we can scare off predators and protect ourselves.

It seems that transgenerational transmissions allow us to pay the dues of the previous generations and to re-establish a form of justice within the clan. The transmission of the emotional stress of a father, a grandmother, or even an uncle may lead to illness in an offspring. The illness will be the solution to an emotional conflict or trauma these relatives could not express or resolve during their lifetime. Their distress and its emotional meaning will then be passed on to the next generation. For instance, an uncle who could not "swallow" the fact that his brother inherited more land than he did after his father's death might predispose a descendant to esophageal disease. A grandmother who could not "digest the filth" related to her husband's affair might program a disease related to the colon in a member of the next generation.

When such conflict still circulates within the clan, healing is often possible through the awareness of such unresolved emotional stress. We can now understand how illness is often rooted at a more innate level than the personal circumstances of an individual during his or her lifetime. It seems none of our circumstances happen by either accident or luck, but in fact are infused by our subconscious, which now allows us to believe that predispositions to certain illnesses can be seen in a different light.

Symbols that are attached to birth, such as the choice of a name, can also influence our lives. Names that are chosen according to religion, tradition, politics, sports, theater, or to honor a deceased member of the clan will remain emotionally charged by the memory and the intention they represent. For instance, a boy named after his brother who died right before the boy's birth might carry a bigger burden of having to *replace the dead child* and never feel good enough for his inconsolable parents. In 2007, I met a young woman called Helen who was named after her grandmother who died when her mother was ten. Helen felt that she somehow took on the role of being the *mother of her mother* by taking care and providing emotional support to her at an early age.

Alejandro Jodorowsky from Chile is a pioneer in Transgenerational Therapy who uses provocative, unusual, and theatrical therapeutic tools to create deep transformation at a clan level. He says that "the subconscious mind is not scientific but it is artistic" and reminds us how we should think of our family tree as a real tree with branches. He states it is possible for organic healing to begin as long as one member of the clan can bring to their consciousness their inherited and subconscious memories of drama, death, injustice, incest, rape, miscarriage, crime, and unfulfilled desires. This will "purify" their memories. According to Jodorowsky, addressing the issues of family members such as parents, aunts, uncles, and grandparents should not be a quest for autonomy and detachment from the clan but rather an opportunity to liberate our ancestors and descendants while healing ourselves in the process (interview of Alejandro Jodorowsky by Patrice Van Eersel, "Your family is a tree inside of you").

Thoughts on German New Medicine

Disease can be compared to a biological emergency measure that increases or decreases the function of an organ in correspondence to an unresolved emotional crisis. Then again, not every individual may have the chance to fully resolve their distress naturally, since it is not always easy to surpass an emotional conflict and life will not necessarily provide an ideal change of circumstances. However, for numerous individuals a resolution can be achieved, whether it is through personal transformation or an environmental change.

During his practice, Dr. Hamer was helping his patients eliminate stress, mainly through what can be called the "practical solution." For instance, Dr. Hamer states he treated a patient who was dying from liver cancer. The patient's distress was related to the "lack of money" he was experiencing after his bank refused to lend him the amount he needed to purchase his dream home. Dr. Hamer personally contacted the bankers in an attempt to convince them to agree to the loan so that the man would be able to resolve his conflict. The bank denied his request, and Dr. Hamer decided that he himself would loan his client the money so that he could buy the house. Dr. Hamer claims his client healed completely without any additional treatment and slowly re-paid his debt to him.

In the above case, Dr. Hamer was able to demonstrate the possible power of the practical solution. Although this type of solution is momentarily strong, it is based on circumstantial changes where one's problem is transferred to others. Ideally, recovery should not be dependent upon modifications coming from other individuals, or simply upon a shift of circumstances. In other words, one person cannot be made responsible for the health of another. True healing comes from a change within oneself.

Since it is our beliefs and not our genes that control our health, how can biological healing last if we keep the same limiting beliefs and perceptions about our issues or traumas? If someone cannot digest a situation, what perception has made them feel they cannot digest it, and how much of that perception is a distortion on their part? How do they filter the world, and what are the subconscious imprints that have predisposed them to such beliefs and perceptions? Aside from any personal impacts, how many are imprints from childhood and how many are directly related to their parents' stresses during gestation, or even belong to their ancestors? How can someone free themselves from those hidden stresses if the environment is perceived as responsible for their misfortune?

If a woman heals breast cancer based on her reconciliation with her partner after he left her for another woman, what is going to happen if one day down the road he has another affair? In order to liberate emotional stress, individuals often need resources that are stronger than just the information about their conflict and its expression in their body. If this woman continues to perceive her husband and his affair in the same way as before, it simply means she did not surpass the problem. However, if she learns how to detach, take responsibility, and manifest emotional independence, she could resolve her struggle for good. In other words, the external problem still exists, but it does not affect her emotionally anymore.

German New Medicine is not a panacea; however, it appears that when individuals have the opportunity to effectively work on their subconscious programs, they can greatly improve their chances to overcome disease.

Cancer is a survival mechanism that prevents the body from expiring quickly from unmanageable stress. It is important to know that if the individual is unsuccessful at resolving the biological conflict in a timely manner, the illness could progress to a point of no return, where healing becomes insurmountable.

Some cancer patients are successfully using methodologies based on Dr. Hamer's findings while incorporating medical treatments intelligently until the conflict resolution is fully completed. When choosing such a path, it is important to be aware of the limitations of Western medicine, which does not validate the two phases of disease nor the presence of brain alterations in the areas corresponding to the affected organs. These modifications (Hamer focuses—"HH"), centered on precise points of the brain, can be identified through a set of concentric rings that can be seen in a computerized tomography scan (CT). These alterations, however, are often considered artifacts by radiologists. According to Dr. Hamer, the location of the focus depends on the nature of the conflict-shock. Although these observations regarding the presence of concentric rings in the brain are contradictory, they also lead to question why the so-called artifacts are always located in the specific area of the brain corresponding to the affected organ. In 1990, the Siemens Corporation (a major manufacturer of CT scanners) officially refuted the presence of concentric rings found on their CT scans as being artifacts.

If we validate the discovery of Dr. Hamer, we can consider that, besides being invasive, treatments such as chemotherapy and radiation can also interfere with the natural process of the healing phase. This is why the ideal situation would be for doctors to consider this new knowledge and incorporate it into their practice.

In the case of certain cancers or other diseases labeled as "incurable," it is essential not to buy into the fear built around a diagnosis but instead ignore definitive "final" statements.

Dr. Hamer's findings will eventually enlighten and change Western medicine views, thus influencing the medical field to base their research on new fundamental principles. It seems there is an amalgam between Dr. Hamer's revolutionary discovery and his therapeutic approach, which might sometimes lack concrete solutions. For the sake of long-term health, the relevance of his findings should not be tainted by the imperfections of some of his results. It goes without saying that in the domain of cancer, Western medicine is no panacea either.

Ultimately, what is important—apart from the biological knowledge—is the art of therapy a practitioner has mastered and the capability to decode and relay information, which cannot be applied to every person in the same way. A combination of knowledge is of the highest importance as well as the ability to intuitively tune into the person's psyche with sensitivity and adaptability toward each different personality. Besides the use of specific powerful tools, it is often this personal interaction that, in essence, unlocks and resolves emotional distress and can ultimately lead to healing.

It is clear that the resistance of Western medicine is also related to many other aspects than just the antithetical concept related to new approaches such as German New Medicine® and Total Biology®. First of all, science is influenced by the philosophy of Descartes and Newton, who dismissed the idea that the mind influences the body. Their visions were that there is no connection between biological matter and the immaterial mind. To complicate matters further, doctors often disregard the reasons some people heal against all odds. They have a tendency to bury the success of such patients under the label of rare cases.

One would think it would be useful to closely study those rare cases in an attempt to decipher what was medically or methodologically different from other cases. Unfortunately, most doctors believe that the mind cannot be more effective than drugs. Similarly, the Germ Theory, which considers germs as invaders and aggressors of the body, is still validated. This scientific theory creates obstacles to exploring the possibility that bacteria are part of our system and stay dormant until our bodies need to use them as optimizers during the healing phase.

These new findings could substantially improve the positive outcome of many illnesses and revolutionize our approach to health.

Most Commonly Asked Questions

If cancer is related to an emotional conflict, why then do smokers develop lung cancer? Aren't cigarettes the cause of such disease?

The emotional conflict related to the fear of death (for oneself, or a loved one) creates at a subconscious level the need for more oxygen in order to improve respiratory function and avoid death. The role of the alveoli in the lung is to acquire oxygen. The meaning of lung cancer, for instance through the proliferation of alveolar cells, is to permit the grasping of more oxygen in order to distribute it to the organs.

Interestingly enough, the behavior of smoking gives an individual the illusion of getting more air in their lungs. Those who smoke give themselves an emotional relief each time they inhale. Ultimately, it is their latent emotional stress that leads them to smoke. One day they might trigger lung cancer because of a conflict shock related to breathing according to their predisposition to the conflict of fear of death (alveoli) or even a conflict linked to the fear of their territory being invaded by someone seen as "the enemy" (bronchi), who might be perceived as "eating up their air."

As always, the conflict might be real, imaginary, virtual, or symbolic, and although cigarettes are metaphorically offering a practical solution to the two subconscious stresses mentioned above, they are not exactly the root cause of the cancer that smokers develop. Just because two elements are simultaneously present in a certain context (in this case smoking and lung cancer) does not mean they are related in the way we anticipate. What is apparent is not always what it seems to be. Notice how Dana Reeve, the wife of Christopher Reeve, although she had never smoked cigarettes, was diagnosed with lung cancer Aug 9, 2005, exactly 10 months after the death of her husband, on Oct 10, 2004. We could ask ourselves how she experienced the traumatic event of her husband's death. Did it create an emotional distress related to the fear of death, leading to lung cancer as an expression of her wanting subconsciously to grasp more oxygen for her husband, who sadly stopped breathing?

What evidence suggests that metastases are not the result of cancer cells migrating from one organ to the other?

If the cause of secondary cancers were related to a spill from primary tumors and an anarchical migration, why would CT scans show a visible mark, indicating the presence of cerebral alterations (Hamer focuses—"HH") in perfect correlation with the primary as well as secondary locations of cancer in the body? We all develop cancerous cells in our body every day. Although the idea that cancer cells can be transported to distant sites has been generally accepted, it has not been proven. All that is known is that cancer cells are present in humans. A Hamer focus systematically manifests in the cerebral relay related to each new affected organ, which clearly indicates a correlation between new stresses and secondary cancers.

According to Dr. Hamer, the reason cancer found in secondary organs has the same histology (cancer type) as the primary one is related to the nature of the initial conflict. If a cancer of the same type is found within other organs, then it is the biological materialization of two shades of the same conflict. In other words, the identity of the original conflict remains present within the expression of another conflict in another organ. Each new cancer is a symbolic solution to a new conflict. For instance, a person with breast cancer (nest conflict) might develop a tumor in the lung (with the same characteristics as the breast tumor) because of her fear of death about her breast cancer.

Is the cause of illness always related to emotional distress? Aren't environmental factors such as pollution, nutritional deficiencies, and toxins also contributing to disease?

The World Health Organization estimates that 20% of deaths in the developing world are attributed to environmental factors, i.e. pollutants, which include lead, mercury, hexavalent chromium, and arsenic. Most often, pollution is held responsible for health issues such as cancer, cognitive impairment, and respiratory problems. The truth is, Western medicine does not know the real cause of cancer. Therefore, practitioners of Western medicine can only blame external factors to create some sort of understanding about cancer. The bottom line is: if pollution were the major cause of cancer, most of us would get sick and not just a small percentage of the population. Cancer existed before the modern world, when the air was still pure and 20th-century pollutants were nonexistent. So what was the cause of cancer then? In reality, it is only when toxicity reaches a level that humans cannot bear that the body will respond through a cellular reaction in order to process and eliminate the excess of poison. During the Chernobyl disaster in Ukraine, most fatalities from the accident were caused by radiation poisoning because toxicity levels were elevated beyond the threshold a human being could absorb. For as long as the level of toxicity can be processed and eliminated by our body, it is unlikely that disease will be triggered (unless a conflict-shock occurs).

Although we are subjected to unhealthy substances, our life span is consistently increasing because we continue to adapt to the environment. Granted, the amount of pollution in big cities is unnatural and unhealthy, but not enough to explain all the different types of cancers. Using the same reasoning, we could also ask ourselves why unhealthy food would be the cause of health issues for some and not for others who eat in an even worse fashion while staying free of disease.

Since there exist reasons to believe that illness is related to emotional conflicts, it is also true that prevention of disease starts with healthy living, including exercise and avoiding sugar, greasy food, alcohol, drugs, and cigarettes. An individual who is depleted energetically will be emotionally unequipped to manage their emotions when caught of guard by a traumatic event, and evidently be more susceptible to a conflict shock. A healthy and conscious lifestyle will certainly promote a strong and balanced mind. A study at Ohio State University demonstrated that women who focused on better nutrition, physical activity, and certain relaxation methods were 68% less likely to die from their cancer in the next eleven years compared to other women who did not improve their lifestyle during and after treatment. Several studies also suggest that emotional states can have an impact on cancer statistics [Andersen et al., 2004, 2008; Blake-Mortimer et al., 1999; Fawzy et al., 1990, 1993; Monti et al., 2006, Spiegel et al., 1989].

The reality is that a better lifestyle can permit an individual to access more resourceful emotional states. An emotional conflict is a matter of perception. A lucid mental state can allow for more understanding towards others and perhaps an ability to let go of the very conflict that is at the root of the illness. Sometimes it is easier to alter our way of looking at an event when we have the support of a healthy mind and body.

Why are some children born with illnesses when they have not yet been exposed to life and stresses?

During the intrauterine period, the fetus is imprinting the emotional conflicts of both parents. A combination of the parents' emotions and their stresses creates an equation. When both parents undergo the same type of stress at the same time, the imprint is even more powerful. The solution to the stress will often emerge instantly through the embryo at a cellular level. A disorder often starts *in utero*, in alignment with the emotions that both parents share. This allows for an immediate biological solution to be expressed through the future offspring. In a peculiar way, the parents' unmanageable stress is alleviated through a download from their brains directly to the embryo's biology. In order to understand this phenomenon, it is important to remember that during pregnancy the survival of the parents prevails (particularly the mother) to insure present and future progeny. The parents' emotional distress is lowered by subconsciously downloading the stress to the embryo.

As an example, one of my clients in Paris came to me for the purpose of improving her relationship with her husband. She had brought her son along with her to the session. He was twelve years old and was born deaf. The woman had always wondered why her son had been afflicted with such condition. I asked her to tell me what had happened during her pregnancy that was related to hearing. It turns out that while being pregnant she had ear infections and did not take care of them properly. When she finally went to a doctor, her infections were so bad that he thought she might lose her hearing. For quite some time, both this woman and her husband feared that she might become deaf.

As always, the brain will express the perfect solution to eliminate stress. If one is on a bike with an intense fear of falling, it will trigger a general discharge of the sympathetic nervous system. Consequently, the brain will need to provide the ultimate solution to interrupt the stress. The solution to the fear of falling off a bike is to actually fall! Once on the ground, the fear of falling no longer exists. In a similar way, during that intense phase of stress related to the fear of becoming deaf, the presence of the embryo provided a way to alleviate this particular fear: it developed an ear impairment and subsequently was born deaf. As Dr. Sabbah would say, "The fear of the thing creates the thing!"

It has been observed that when the parents have the same distress at the same time, the child might be born with a biological expression that corresponds precisely to the emotional conflict with which both parents struggled. However, if only one parent has a conflict, then a related disease might manifest later on in the offspring's life.

Why do our animals get sick?

Domesticated animals can develop illnesses related to their owner's stresses whether real, imaginary, virtual, or symbolic. A pet does, in fact, act as an extension of its master's brain, absorbing its owner's distress like a sponge and expressing the related illness. It is almost as if the animal's sensitivity and devotion elicits a transfer of the emotional struggle of its master into its own biology, thereby materializing illness within itself instead. For instance, a female dog might suffer from ovarian cancer after her owner experienced the profound loss of her daughter.

What is the cause of mental illness?

Dr. Hamer presented new concepts about the cause behind mental illnesses and the cerebral phenomenon that can trigger psychoses, such as depression, schizophrenia, autism, and so forth. The source of mental illness appears to be related to the presence of two or more active conflicts and their Hamer focuses (HH) in specific areas of the brain. Autism, for example, is the result of the constellation of two Hamer focuses in the cerebral cortex, one located on the larynx mucosa relay and the other on the stomach/pancreas duct relay.

The thesis presented by Dr. Hamer is unprecedented and, because of his findings, so much about illness can now be reevaluated, including mental disorders. According to research, mental illnesses are the result of genetic vulnerabilities and exposure to environmental stressors. The key revealed by Dr. Hamer is that multiple emotional conflicts can create constellations in the brain and cause mental disorders. Those constellations can now be located through CT scans for acute diagnoses. One day, besides antidepressants, antipsychotics, and mood stabilizers, new solutions may emerge as a result of the understanding of this new paradigm.

Isn't Western medicine progressing and helping more and more cancer patients?

Although billions of dollars are given to research, we can observe the escalation of cancer deaths. What does that mean? For as long as Western medicine keeps the same paradigm about the origin of cancer and only recognizes surgery, chemotherapy, radiation, and immunotherapy, a breakthrough is unlikely to arise. Unfortunately, humongous financial amounts are allocated to such favored forms of treatment. It is obvious that modern medicine is not on the right track to curing cancer; otherwise, the results stemming from the research would improve. In addition to the augmentation of human emotional conflicts and distress, due to the pressures of modern lifestyle, the notion of cancer itself creates stress and continues to strike fear. This is true when we observe the stress women over the age of forty repeatedly experience when they undergo their annual mammograms.

Cancer rates have been climbing steadily in the US since 1940, in synchronicity with the increase use of screening tests. Research published July 9, 2009, in the *British Medical Journal* reveals that as many as one in every three breast cancers diagnosed by mammogram screening would never have become life threatening and could naturally have regressed on its own, without treatment. Could the increase in the cancer rate be related to medical conduct of over-diagnoses of imaging resources to detect tumors that were not actually malignant?

What happens, then, when healthy individuals are thrown in the category of cancer patients and subjected to painful and toxic treatments? Could some early deaths be related to such unnecessary extreme therapies and not cancer itself?

An article in the *Los Angeles Times* (Christie Aschwanden Aug. 17, 2009) reveals "autopsy studies have found undetected breast cancer in about 37% of women who died from other causes. And a study of 42,238 Norwegian women calculated that 22% of symptom free cancers found on screening mammograms naturally regressed on their own."

When considering the theory of Dr. Hamer, we may understand why cancer can regress on its own, since it is related to an emotional distress that can be resolved. Radiologists and oncologists would interpret scans and mammograms very differently if they were made aware of the two phases of disease. At the same time, individuals would be protected from unnecessary threat, the ultimate invasion of their bodies, and the subsequent psychological impacts.

Cancer is on the rise in alignment with conscious and subconscious expectations most individuals now have, that cancer will hit them one day. The threat of cancer, its magnitude, and its unstoppable progression bombard us on a daily basis. In particular, the "pink ribbon" campaign for breast cancer has taken on a life of its own, along with the astounding amount of "pink" paraphernalia being sold on behalf of these charities. It almost seems that with "Cancer Awareness" walks/runs and so on, cancer is indeed accepted as a fact of life and thus becomes a self-fulfilling prophecy. We all know of someone who has died of cancer, and the fear related to it is so ingrained within the population that, for most, when cancer appears in their body, it might as well be a death sentence.

For some a "do it yourself proposition" is the only option left and opens doors to the danger of unreliable "cancer cures." Dr. Hamer's discovery about disease does not constitute a cure. It is a set of findings that could lead to overcoming illness. If scientists and researchers would accept the idea that the cells of our bodies are affected by our thoughts and accordingly modify their approach to illness, a new style of mind-therapy could be further developed and incorporated. This would result in a form of treatment that would respect the laws of nature and promote emotional as well physical health.

The Future

---

*To heal, it is necessary and sufficient to remove
the source of conflict within one's self.*
CARL G. JUNG

One day both German New Medicine and Western medicine may possibly combine their efforts to further understand and treat illness, and we might witness the emergence of a new style of medicine that will combine modalities for emotional healing with adequate remedies. In the meantime, healing will continue to manifest and increase, since more individuals will access a new awareness and benefit from the findings of Dr. Hamer, Dr. Sabbah, Dr. Marc Frechet, and Anne Ancelin Shützenberger, among many others. We are living in one of the most fascinating eras of humankind where brilliant new knowledge regarding illness is finally surfacing and is being made available to everyone.

I hope this information has given you insight, changed your opinion about disease, and alleviated some fears you might have. Perhaps now you can look at your life as an unfolding scenario where you have the power to modify any aspect of it. Always remember that when something unpleasant happens to you, it is possible for you to change your perception and even search for a way in which a challenging time might be a blessing in disguise!

I hope you are inspired and become independent of opinions you might have been programmed to believe. That is the first step to healing.

How wonderful to realize we can create health from within.

With passion,
Isabelle Benarous

SUGGESTED READING

The Summary of the New Medicine, Dr. Ryke Geerd Hamer
www.newmedicine.ca

Recall Healing: Unlocking the Secrets of Illness, Gilbert Renaud, Ph.D.
www.recallhealing.com

The Scientific Chart of German New Medicine, Dr. Ryke Geerd Hamer
www.newmedicine.ca

The Ancestor Syndrome, Anne Ancelin Schützenberger, Routledge

Biology of Belief, Bruce H. Lipton Ph.D., Hay House Inc.

Biogenealogy: Decoding the Psychic Roots of Illness, Patrick Obissier,
Healing Arts Press

*The Journey: A Practical Guide to Healing Your Life and Setting Yourself
Free,* Brandon Bays, Fireside

INDEX

ABOUT THE AUTHOR

Isabelle Benarous is a Trainer of Neuro-Linguistic Programming and a specialist in the field of Total Biology® and German New Medicine®. She is an expert in the psychology of change and specializes in the resolution of emotional distress leading to disease. Fundamental discoveries have been made in Europe by researchers who show that illness is the result of a shock, hence leading to an emotional crisis. Each organ in the body can potentially express such emotional disturbance through cellular changes and therefore disease. The seriousness of a condition is proportional to the amount of stress related to the shock, trauma, or chronic struggle. Illnesses such as cancer can now be understood through a new paradigm that can permit individuals to directly take control of their health through self-awareness and perceptual changes.

This book will permit the reader to discover the undeniable logic of an unprecedented approach regarding the mind-body connection. It will also reveal new hypotheses regarding ancestral impacts as well as in utero distress and the type of effects they can produce in one's life.

Isabelle Benarous developed the method of Bio-Reprogramming®, which permits the identification of emotional conflicts while utilizing a wide spectrum of tools to provide individuals with concrete and powerful solutions to achieve emotional healing. As a Therapist and Trainer, her approach is combining German New Medicine®, Total Biology®, Neuro-Linguistic-Programming, and Ericksonian Hypnosis among other modalities.

Isabelle Benarous is bringing to this field the strength and knowledge developed during her personal experience with illness as she helped a loved one, who remarkably benefited from her deep understanding and commitment to this type of approach. She has been introducing the concept of Biological Decoding in United States since 2001. Currently, she maintains a private practice at the Healing Arts Center of Altadena in Southern California as well as conducting seminars throughout the United States and Europe.

www.bioreprogramming.net

email: info@bioreprogramming.net